Given to .

with al

for the author .

NATIONAL INSTITUTE SOCIAL SERVICES LIBRARY NO. 41

TOWARDS DEATH WITH DIGNITY

National Institute Social Services Library

Towards Death with Dignity

Caring for Dying People

SYLVIA POSS

London
GEORGE ALLEN & UNWIN
Boston   Sydney

GEORGE ALLEN & UNWIN LTD
40 Museum Street, London WC1A 1LU

British Library Cataloguing in Publication Data

Poss, Sylvia
    Towards death with dignity. – (National Institute
social services, no. 41)
    1. Terminal care
    I. Title
    362.1   R726.8

    ISBN 0–04–362041–8
    ISBN 0–04–362042–6 Pbk

Set in 10 on 11 point Times by Grove Graphics, Tring
and printed in Great Britain
by Billing and Sons Ltd., Guildford, London
and Worcester

CONTENTS

For Dr Reginald Hegy
whose inspiration gave birth to this work

THE PURPOSE OF LIFE
Enid Henke

———◆———

A friend and I were considering life and its purpose. I said, even with increasing paralysis and loss of speech, I believed there was a purpose for my life but I was not sure what it was at that particular time. We agreed to pray about it for a week: I was then sure that my present purpose is simply to receive other people's prayers and kindness and to link together all those who are lovingly concerned about me, many of whom are unknown to one another. After a while my friend said, 'It must be hard to be the wounded Jew when by nature you would rather be the Good Samaritan'.

It is hard: it would be unbearable were it not for my belief that the wounded man and the Samaritan are inseparable. It was the helplessness of the one that brought out the best in the other and linked them together.

In reflecting on the parable I am particularly interested in the fact that we are not told the wounded man recovered. I have always assumed that he did but it now occurs to me that even if he did not recover the story would still stand as a perfect example of true neighborliness [*sic*]. You will remember that the story concludes with the Samaritan asking the innkeeper to take care of the man, but he assures him of his own continuing interest and support: so the innkeeper becomes linked.

If, as my friend suggested, I am cast in the role of the wounded man, I am not unmindful of the modern day counterparts of the priest and Levite, but I am overwhelmed by the kindness of so many 'Samaritans'. There are those who, like you, have been praying for me for a long time and constantly reassure me of continued interest and support. There are others who have come into my life – people I would never have met had I not been in need who are now being asked to take care of me. I like to think that all of us have been linked together for a purpose which will prove a means of blessing to us all. (Henke, 1972).

This statement was dictated with some difficulty because of a speech defect by a young woman who was dying of a progressive paralysis. It was finished two weeks before she died, after four years of illness.

Permission to reprint this statement in its entirety came from Dr C. Saunders, St Christopher's Hospice. London, November 1975.

PREFACE

The recent explosion of literature on the once taboo topic of death and dying tells us that we, contemporary men and women, feel uncomfortable in our confrontation with death, and require help in adjusting to it. Despite the wealth of new writings on the topic, however, no book on the social worker's standpoint has yet appeared. With this volume I am hoping to fill the gap. My ideas are the outcome of my research and experience of social work in the terminal care field. It is written for all the members of the health care team and for dying persons and their relatives, although my emphasis remains a social work perspective.

This book offers both my own ideas and the work of a host of previous writers, for example, Kübler-Ross, Saunders, Schoenberg *et al.*, Burton, Abrams, Hinton, Brim *et al.*, and Weisman, among others. I am indebted to them all. In suggesting how we may help people who are dying. I have attempted to provide a theoretical background by synthesising the ideas and work of many previous writers and then linking them with my own observations. This book is thus intended as a practical guide for terminal care workers.

My contribution to the already considerable literature on terminal care has to do with both the psychosocial and the spiritual care of the dying person. Although the book remains essentially a social work text, I offer a dual perspective of the situation: an integrated view, combining my spiritual and social work knowledge. My personal motivation for work in the field of terminal care lies in the certain knowledge of life after death, and my own experience that God helps where no man can. Nevertheless, this book has not been easy to write. There are no absolute answers as to how to care for the dying person. One idea has been tried after the other – as much in the care of the patient as in the writing of this book. The outcome represents my present state of thinking. There have been long periods of intense effort with no apparent results. It has often been a temptation to abandon the task altogether. Staying with it has taken perseverance, commitment and a rethinking of the whole project. The only way I have been able to use these struggles creatively has been to hold on to them, to keep me in touch with some of the thoughts and feelings that accompany caring for the dying patient and the process of dying itself. The feelings have thus been valuable, if painful.

A further difficulty in writing has come from the soul-searching question of whether I need to be an expert in order to teach others. For a long time I held the unrealistic expectation of having all the answers. It was only in the intense struggle of formulating my ideas on teamwork (Chapter 7) that I came to the painful realisation that I did not have complete foolproof guidelines to offer to readers – and did not need to hold up the completion of the task until I had found or compiled them.

The outcome, this book on terminal care, is not confined to the social worker, but is intended for all whose work brings them into contact with people who are approaching death: dying persons themselves, nurse, doctor, chaplain, paramedical staff, colleagues in the community – for example, health visitor and district nurse, general practitioner, employer, teacher and lawyer. Hopefully, it will also be of use to the layman, relative, neighbour or friend who after several decades of avoiding contact with dying is once again increasingly being called upon to be involved in some way in the death of his fellow man. Hence although the underlying foundation is a social work base, the term 'caregiver' will be used to denote the person – whether lay or professional – who is tending the dying patient. Competence to do the task is important, irrespective of original training or profession.

Nor is another new specialisation implied. The terminal care expert, who absolves every other caregiver of the responsibility, makes a mockery of the whole concept of dying as a natural life event. The aim of sound terminal caring is to reinforce its place in the community, in ordinary homes where family members can, with some facilitative help or basic training, be enabled to manage the task of tending a dying relative for themselves. This view sets terminal care in its context as one of many integral aspects of several professions – medicine, nursing, theology, social work, and so on. All these service professions need to care both for people who are likely to recover, and for those who are not. Thus terminal care work, if it is to succeed in its task of total patient care and contributing to the health and welfare of the whole community, encompasses all the methods of social work. Some of them – social group work, supervision/consultation, administration and research – will not be focused on in this book as their application is, I believe, no different in this setting from any other field of social work.

This book will, however, focus on three of social work's major methods: social casework, community work and teaching. The lists of tasks outlined for the social worker to undertake are numerous and lengthy. They may well seem impossible to accomplish. I therefore want to stress that they have been included not because they all need to be undertaken, but in order to sketch the scope of the work and help the worker in difficulty to identify the area from which her problems may stem. I do not mean to imply that any one social worker should be undertaking all these activities herself. The community work section, in particular, is included to draw attention to the need for this social work method in the field of terminal care, and to alert medical social work practitioners who may be involved only in direct patient care and who may omit to consider these aspects of the terminal situation. Whether the same social worker should attempt both clinical work and community work simultaneously is an issue for debate. Both advantages and disadvantages appear to prevail. On the one hand she has an ideal position, from her first-hand contact with the individual patient, to prescribe what community facilities are needed. On the other hand, the energising anger that is often appropriate for mobilising community enthusiasm and activity is likely to infiltrate her efforts with her individual patient in a non-therapeutic way.

Another issue that merits debate is whether to refer to the dying person as a 'patient', a term which denotes sickness and, within the medical model, abnormality. If dying is to be viewed as a natural life process, and on that thesis this book rests, it may be important to regard the dying individual as a person rather than a patient. (Do we need reminding that every patient is a person?) Since the dying person often suffers an illness prior to death, and so may be a patient, the terms have been used interchangeably in the text. The point to emphasise is that it may be crucial for the medical caregivers to acknowledge a point in time when each patient becomes a (dying) person once more – that is, a time when their goal needs to change from the cure of a patient to the care of a *person* who is unlikely to recover.

ACKNOWLEDGEMENTS

I am gratefully indebted to many people and institutions for guidance and assistance offered while this project was in progress.

Because of the particular demands involved in working with dying persons, I wish first to acknowledge the Divine Help and Strength which made the entire venture possible.

Four supervisors influenced the original study on which this book is based. The late Professor Felix Brümmer, Professor Ceceil Muller, Dr Annemie de Vos and Dr Yvonne Blake each made different, valuable contributions to my thinking, and to the final outcome of the project. Since then, many of my ideas have changed as my experience has broadened. New thoughts and valued critical comments have come from my publisher and his reviewers in the form of penetrating assessments of my third and fourth drafts.

During the course of rendering a social work service to fifty dying patients and their families, I relied heavily on the support of the clinical consultant to the study, Dr Yvonne Blake. Her steady interest has been a major factor in enabling me to complete what has been a difficult but rewarding undertaking.

The University of the Witwatersrand facilitated the completion of the research project by granting me leave privileges, and the Human Sciences Research Council provided a financial grant for the study. The Director of the Transvaal Department of Hospital Services and the Superintendent of the Johannesburg Hospital gave permission for research to be conducted in that hospital.

This book could not have materialised without the participation of the patients involved, now deceased, and their families. It was not easy for them to accommodate a research project while in the midst of personal suffering and tragedy. Their motive for co-operating so willingly was not infrequently the wish that others in a similar position might benefit as a result. I share their wish.

In the course of rendering the service, many demands were made on personnel in private and hospital practice who were involved in the care of the patients in question. Especial thanks go to Mr P. Marchand, principal thoracic surgeon, and Drs R. V. Dando and R. Saner, consultant physicians, Chemotherapy Subdepartment, Johannesburg Hospital, from whom the majority of patients were referred.

Dr Cecily Saunders of London, Dr Elisabeth Kübler-Ross of Flossmoor, Illinois, and Mrs Ruth Abrams of Boston all gave generously of their ideas and sent valuable reprints of their own articles.

Many friends helped: Dr Mary Edginton, Iain McNeill, Dr Wilma

Hoffman, Irene Comaroff and Anthony Wolbarst all read and commented on various drafts. Professor Paul Hare and Dr Peter Cusins were particularly instrumental in facilitating the work on the final drafts.

Mrs M. Nell, Mrs Arlene Schwartz and Ms Tibbie Ferreira typed successive drafts of this manuscript.

My friends and family and my sister, Dorothy, showed untiring support and patience while the task achieved completion.

Part One

APPROACHING DEATH:
THE TERMINAL CRISIS

Chapter 1

—————◆—————

BACKGROUND

One view of man assumes that each life-phase constitutes a challenge to the individual and that the human being is ready to move on to a further stage of life only once the work of the preceding stage has been completed. (Towle, 1945; Eric Erikson, 1950; Caplan, 1970.) Even though death may interrupt the life-cycle at any stage, dying constitutes the final stage of human development and as such may be perceived as part of a natural, developmental continuum of life (Weisman and Kastenhaum, 1968). Since death is natural, it is possible, as in the mastery of other life-crises, for the individual to use his dying as an opportunity to develop emotionally and spiritually. Ideally, growth in the dying person lies both in working towards a dignified death (Saunders, 1976) and in preparing for life after death (Autton, 1969; and Dominian, 1970).

The effort involved in such growth may be referred to synonymously as 'dying work', 'death work' or 'terminal crisis work'. These terms denote the mental, emotional, social and spiritual work required of the patient in order to come to terms with dying and death, and so to die with dignity. As the helping professions have assimilated the term of 'mourning work', and Lindemann's (1944) definition of 'grief work', the term 'work' is used throughout the text in order to indicate that a great deal of energy and effort are required to resolve the crisis involved in dying. Hence the patient cannot master the terminal crisis, that is, he cannot die with dignity, until his dying work has been completed. 'Dignified dying' and 'acceptance of death' will be used synonymously to indicate the optimal outcome of dying work completed. It should be noted that death with dignity implies death with physical, emotional and spiritual dignity.

A discussion of whether life actually continues after death falls beyond the scope of this book. Many studies, however, have provided evidence which has led investigators to conclude that life does in fact continue after death (Osler, 1906; Lodge, 1925; Conan Doyle, 1926; Osis, 1961; Barrett, 1962 and Hegy, 1964). Whether the caregiver believes in a life after death or not, Carlozzi (1968) stresses that the terminal patient needs to be prepared for life, death, and life after death. Like me, many people believe that man is immortal. I will therefore consider the implications which this conviction holds for the various participants in the terminal situation: patient, relatives, those who tend the patient and particularly the social worker. If, in fact, life does not continue after death, nothing will have been lost by adopting this standpoint. If, on the other hand, existence is continued beyond the grave, in whatever form, preparation for it will have constituted an appropriate 'life-task'. For my atheist readers or patients, this approach will be easily enough modified. Similarly, whether the patient grows in stature or not will depend, in part, on how he has managed other life situations. In this sense the way he approaches death is likely to reflect his manner in life.

Preparation for death may well be necessary, but who is the best person to offer such help to the patient? It is my firm contention that many people – both lay and professional – hold strategic positions from which to aid the patient in his final life struggle. The family's claim naturally takes precedence. In the absence of willing relatives, social work, because of its strong psychosocial orientation to life, is one such profession. But it cannot manage the task alone. Many disciplines need to be involved in terminal care. No one profession holds the monopoly of such care. Hence whatever social work service is rendered, it is always offered in relation to the rest of a caring team.

The broad scope of such a therapeutic team reveals the emergent need for designating one of its members as 'primary caregiver', namely, that person who will, on behalf of the entire team, carry out the major part of the psychosocial and spiritual work involved in facilitating the patient's resolution of the terminal crisis. In this sense the doctor in charge may or may not be the primary caregiver; he nevertheless retains responsibility for the patient's total care. Abrams (1974) distinguishes a primary family caregiver from a primary professional caregiver, and defines a primary family caregiver as 'some-one (i.e. a relative) emotionally close to the patient . . . the physician's closest ally.'

Unless otherwise stated, this book is written from the point of view of the social worker as primary professional caregiver in the terminal situation. It is however not my intention to suggest that the social worker routinely does or should fill this role. On the contrary, wherever possible the family should be supported in this role. Where that is not possible, the doctor, nurse, or chaplain, to name but a few, will all at times fill a similar role in terminal care. Other people who might make up such a team are likely to include the patient, his relatives, doctors, nurses, social worker, chaplain, volunteer, paramedical staff, laboratory technicians, dietician, radiotherapists and other medical specialists in the hospital. In the community the homecare team may include the dying person, his family, general practitioner, public health nurse, district nurse, friends, neighbours, volunteers, teacher or employer, and parish priest.

MOTIVATION FOR TERMINAL CARE WORK

Many health professionals have acknowledged difficulties in their work with dying people. To the physician the patient often represents failure; to the nurse, a futile and depressing case; to the family, frequently, a financial burden; and to his friends, clergyman, social worker and employer, an uncomfortable obligation. Why then work in this traumatic field? What, anyway, is the point of growth in the face of impending death? To those who have asked these questions, I suggest that this work is worth doing, for the benefit of both the patient and ourselves, the caregivers. For example, health and welfare work is concerned not only with the preservation of life, but also with enhancing the quality of that life, even in dying. The motivation for it rests, then, in the belief that the patient's task in the final life-phase, dying, can be a positive, fulfilling accomplishment. It is true that work in this area may not appear to yield lasting, tangible results; nor can rehabilitation or cure be achieved. Nevertheless, it is the quality of life that matters, not its quantity; time is relative. The emphasis in terminal care is not, therefore, on time *per se*, but on the best use of such time as may be available. No accomplishment is negated by its completion; nor is life negated because it is about to end, or begin anew. Consequently the mandate for caring stands: to help the dying person to reach a contemplative integration of his life by way of its completion. In so doing the patient will have accomplished growth, integration and fulfilment akin to the development of earlier life-phases. In addition, if life after death is a reality growth while dying takes on proportions of eternal significance and, indeed, demands our vital attention.

Another reason for terminal care work is that benefits from work with dying patients accrue both to patients and to those who care for them. In helping others to die with dignity we, the caregivers, are in a position to witness the dignity inherent in a life that is ending. Since 'a dignified death proclaims the significance of all men' (Fulton, 1966), we are assured of the dignity of all life, and reassured of our own dignity in both living and dying. Conversely, the conviction that it is possible for man to die with dignity carries encouragement for patients and caregivers alike, as it enables us to remain in close contact with the suffering and loss that dying entails. The more people experience a patient's achievements in dying, the more they will all be able to help others – and themselves – in all sorts of situations which involve endings.

At the same time, an international climate of renewed interest in the fields of dying, death, bereavement, suicide and terminal care invites

Table 1.1 A Framework for Social Work in Terminal Care

SOCIAL WORK IN TERMINAL CARE

PURPOSE: TO FACILITATE THE RESOLUTION OF THE DYING PERSON'S CRISIS (that is, through the accomplishment of certain tasks)*
METHOD: THE SOCIAL WORK HELPING/CHANGE PROCESS (with individuals, groups and communities)

Social Work service category Part II	Social Work functions Part II	*Social Work tasks (Chapters 6 and 7)	Social Science and Social Work knowledge	Social Work practice skill areas
A Direct work: working with dying persons and their relatives, individually and in groups (Chapter 6)	I Terminal crisis work (Chapter 6)	i facilitating the patient's progress through successive emotional stages of adjustment to death	the nature of the terminal crisis and its resolution } Chapters 2, 3 and 4	i assessing problems
		ii responding to the terminal patient's growing awareness of his condition		ii collecting data
		iii aiding the patient to balance hope and fear	psychology of dying	iii making initial contacts
		iv facilitating the reversal and relinquishing processes involved in terminal adjustment		iv negotiating contracts
		v ensuring unimpeded detachment from human relationships	sociology of death-related behaviour	v forming action systems
		vi providing a climate in which spiritual issues may be explored		vi maintaining and co-ordinating action systems
		vii terminal crisis work with the family of the dying person	selected aspects of medical sociology	vii exercising influence
		viii facilitating the patient/family's decision with regard to the extraordinary prolongation of life	citizen and consumer participation in terminal care programmes (Chapter 7)	viii terminating the change effort
		ix aiding bereaved relatives with their grief work		
	II Environmental Management (tangible service) (Chapter 6)	i planning where terminal care can best be offered	community resources and facilities organisational aspects of institutions	
B Working with significant others (Chapter 7)	III Interpretive work between social work and the health disciplines (Chapter 7)	i initiating open communication for terminal care work	multidisciplinary teamwork (Chapter 7)	
		ii aiding the caregiving team to decide in which awareness context each terminal patient should be cared for	social policies and structures at national, regional, and local levels	
		iii decoding the patient's behaviour	human growth and development	

family dynamics
communications theory
adult education principles
systems theory
learning theory
crisis intervention
social work administration
numerous theories regarding individual, group, and community processes of social work help/change efforts, including social casework (Chapter 6) social group work (Chapter 7) social work and community organisation and development (Chapter 7)

} (Chapter 5)

In addition, the ability to tolerate close contact with dying and death and the ability to take an active social work role in terminal care

iv ensuring the designation of a primary care-giver
v focusing on the feelings which colleagues experience in relation to their work
vi guiding colleagues in the selection and referral of terminal patients for social work intervention
vii participating in decisions concerning the extraordinary prolongation of life

IV Community work
(Chapter 7)

i allocating formal responsibility for the care of the terminal patient to an authoritative body in the health care system
ii developing terminal care service facilities in the community
iii developing training facilities for terminal care workers
iv ensuring continuity in the care of the terminal patient (that is, influencing social policy towards comprehensive health care)
v educating a death-denying society concerning terminal care issues
vi including consumer and citizen participation in the decisions concerning dying, and the planning and provision of terminal care facilities

V Education
(Chapter 7)

i planning each training event as an adult education exercise
ii facilitating the learner's participation in each phase of the learning cycle
iii linking the current learning process with the processes under discussion: caring and dying

C Activities to enhance the quality of the service
(That is, indirect service to patients)

VI Administrative work associated with the total service

VII Supervisory and/or consultative work

VIII Study of relevant Literature

No social work tasks specific to terminal care work

further research into these areas, particularly so in communities where relatively little study has, as yet, been attempted in these fields. Despite the great increase in awareness of and interest in the topics of dying and death displayed by allied disciplines, recent social work literature has reported relatively little and isolated research into terminal care, the dying person and the role of the social worker in this field. As a profession committed to the quality of all life-stages, social work's neglect of this aspect of living requires redress. Hence this book is being attempted.

A FRAMEWORK FOR SOCIAL WORK PRACTICE

Thinking about social work in terminal care may be facilitated by a framework which enables the reader to see at a glance, step by step, what is involved and what she can do in this field. Table 1.1 serves as a guide both to the book and to her work. The framework, which leans on selected aspects of Pincus and Minahan's (1973) model for theoretical support, consists of parameters essential to any model for social work practice: values, sanctions, knowledge, principles, purpose, functions, tasks, skills, method and process. Together these elements constitute a dynamic, interrelated, functioning unit, linked by relationships and bonded by a common purpose. People in relationship to each other form systems in which the framework operates. It should thus be noted that much of the terminal care helping process portrayed statically in Table 1.1 is in fact intangible, dynamic and complicated.

The model may be read, first, as a summary of the book and a suggested framework for practice within which the social worker can move around. It may be frequently consulted, to serve as a checklist or way of monitoring one's comprehension. And it can be returned to at the completion of the book, to reinforce what has been learnt. Thereafter it serves as a one-page guide to the practitioner.

The framework is made up of content both from within this book and from the wider fields of social science and social work knowledge. The specific content of terminal care work is provided here; the methods of applying this content remain those of social work in all fields. Thus the reader may be reassured: no new methodology or profession is needed to do terminal care work, while this book will introduce her to the new content which she will be required to bring to such work. But since increasing knowledge does not necessarily lessen the social worker's apprehension, especially in this field, it is understandable that many workers will feel apprehensive of terminal care work until they have developed some skill in it. The skills required will therefore be discussed in a later chapter. Hopefully, reading this book will play some part in equipping the worker who feels anxious about her task.

With the generic-specific continuum in mind, note then that this terminal care model rests mainly upon a medical social work foundation (Butrym, 1967, p. 10). In other words, it is in *content* that social work in terminal care differs from social work practice in other fields. At the same time it is important to remember that work with a person who is dying may be undertaken from any setting, and not only within the medical field. The content of social work in terminal care takes the form of a response to the terminal crisis. It is viewed as a response because the inevitability of death precludes the prevention of the terminal situation. Once it develops, however, it presents a mandate to the caregivers to respond, in order to ensure that the person may continue to live, and then to die, with dignity.

The social work tasks which have been formulated in the model constitute the 'what' of the service. As such, they highlight the specialised content of social work in terminal care. Similarly, the purpose, functions, tasks and skills specified within the model imply an understanding of the nature of the terminal crisis, for which additional knowledge is required and which this book provides. The other elements in the model are common to all fields of social work practice. The social work functions listed in the framework take most effect when executed in a social work context including some generic activities to enhance the quality of the service, for example, social work education, administrative work, supervision and/or consultation and a study of relevant literature. Hence the last three functions appear in the framework but merit no further discussion in this text.

As it stands, the model offers some qualitative components of terminal care work. Its proportions have not been formulated, and cannot be prescribed. All the elements listed are essential, in proportions to be worked out in each specific service. Some proportions are however suggested here, purely as a guide:

(1) With regard to the frequency with which each social work function is likely to feature in a total service to the dying person and his family, terminal crisis work (that is, direct, clinical work) is likely to feature as the single major function in the service. Environmental management is required considerably less in terminal care than in many other fields of social work, where direct, tangible services form a major proportion of the total service. Administrative work associated with the total service is likely to form the major indirect social work function, constituting a proportion somewhat smaller than terminal crisis work. Interpretive work between social work and the health disciplines is likely to constitute an increasing proportion of the total service, as social workers gain in skill and confidence in their contribution to terminal care work. Community work, in a patient-centred service, remains a minor social function. In a community-centred ser-

vice, however, it would form a major function. Consultation, or supervision, remains a vital aspect of any social work service in terminal care. The needs of the worker are likely to dictate the frequency with which this activity will feature in the total service.

Thus both direct work and activities on the dying person's behalf are essential to the total service and, as suggested by Pincus and Minahan's (1973) theoretical framework, it is possible to predict that functions undertaken in indirect service to the patient are likely to constitute a greater proportion of the total service than direct, clinical work with the dying person/family.

(2) With reference to the intensity of the social work service, it may be assumed that fairly intensive social work intervention is required if the service is to fulfil its aim. At the same time, however, it is important to note that non-intensive service to dying persons and their families may also be positively experienced. Minimal social work intervention, carefully timed, can prove effective. In the light of the present scarcity of social welfare resources, this form of social work aid should not be overlooked. In particular, several groups of patients are likely to benefit from such non-intensive social work intervention. For example:

passive people, who would not ordinarily acknowledge their need of help, who would be unlikely to seek help for themselves and who would be unlikely to use regular help in an active way were it available to them. But if such help were offered to them in a non-threatening way and they were reminded of its availability, they would be likely to accept and use it once they admitted some limited need or asked for something specific;

patients who are *denying* their plight will see no need of regular social work help, but may request some specific practical aid, if the need arises, (for example, for homecare arrangements);

patients who are *resistant* to social work intervention, on account of previous encounters with 'the welfare' may welcome some limited, short-term support over particularly traumatic periods in the terminal situation;

patients who *cope* while they have sufficient resources in their families, communities and themselves to draw on may nevertheless benefit from infrequent, supportive contact with a social worker. Such a service is likely to include information giving, assurance that the family's level of coping is adequate and reassurance of the availability of further help, should it be needed.

In short, time-limited, problem-focused, non-intensive social work is likely to prove an acceptable form of intervention to those patients who have some difficulty in acknowledging their need of help and in asking for help. Such help is likely to be fairly practical and short-term, or, in some circumstances, may be worded in practical terms to disguise a deeper, often unacknowledged need. Non-intensive social work service may effectively take the form of both counselling and/or environmental management – but offered in a negotiated, contractual way, so that each contact is fairly self-contained. Each interview therefore contains both diagnostic and therapeutic elements.

(3) The number of dying persons who are likely to require work in each separate social work function will probably vary. It may be assumed that the majority of terminal patients are likely to require interpretive work on their behalf, terminal crisis work and associated administrative work (that is, one function from each of the categories of service in the framework). On the other hand, relatively few dying persons are likely to require that all the social work functions formulated for terminal care work are in fact undertaken on their behalf. The above observations should not be allowed to mask the value of community work and supervision/consultation, two social work functions through which progress made *vis-à-vis* one particular person is likely to benefit other people also, without necessitating further efforts on the worker's part.

A framework for social work in terminal care has been formulated. Concerning concepts, analytical frameworks and the models built on them, Pincus and Minahan (1973) state that

These are abstractions from our empirical knowledge base, and represent ways to view, think about, and organize knowledge. Concepts cannot be referred to as right or wrong. Rather we speak of them in terms of how useful they are in serving their purpose. (p. 38)

In similar vein, this framework for social work in terminal care should not be viewed as right or wrong but, hopefully, as useful in guiding future practitioners in this and allied settings. It is not presented as a blueprint and will therefore require modification according to the specific circumstances in which it is to be applied. It may however be seen as a confirmation of the commonly held view that social work does indeed have a contribution to make to the care of the dying person, the absence of a clear definition of which has to date prevented its realisation (Spoor, 1975).

Chapter 2

ADJUSTMENT TO THE PROSPECT OF DEATH

Crisis theory has alerted us to the work that people have to do for themselves in order to master any life crises (Rapoport, 1963b). Dying, life's terminal crisis, is no exception. It demands a great deal of work – physical, social, spiritual, intellectual and emotional – on the part of the dying person if death is to be achieved with peace and dignity. Some of this work is likely to be undertaken consciously, while much of it may remain at an unconscious or non-verbal level. If we, the caregivers, have a full appreciation of what this complicated situation involves and of what the patient has to endure it will equip us for the task of enabling him to reach his goal. It goes without saying that the person who is dying will have far greater work to do if he has to accomplish it against a background of physical pain, and personal humiliation. Where sound medical care and efficient and dignified pain control are not present he may need to use all his waning energy in these physical spheres and have very little left with which to work on the 'luxuries' of his psychosocial and spiritual adjustment to death.

What then does the patient have to do by way of preparation in order to accept impending death? Several views exist. Unless otherwise stated, the ideas in this chapter come from Dr Elisabeth Kübler-Ross (1970a, 1970b and 1972). She suggests that the patient's adjustment work involves progressing through a sequence of normal, healthy emotional stages, from the onset of the illness to death itself. They are: denial, isolation, anger, bargaining, depression and then acceptance. Although each stage is to be discussed separately, it should be noted that each one may vary in duration, recur, or overlap as ambivalence, depending on whether that emotion has been thoroughly worked through, integrated, or not.

THE FIRST RESPONSE: DENIAL

Denial is a radical but almost universal response to a grave medical shock. It is more usually needed at the beginning of a serious illness than towards the end of life. Later on the need fluctuates. It is often therefore a temporary response to the awareness of terminal illness. Denial is a healthy initial reaction to any uncomfortable and painful situation, as it allows the patient time to mobilise other more adaptive strategies. Ideally, denial slowly gives way to defences which enable the patient to confront the situation, rather than forcing him to avoid the difficulty. But because the situation *is* a difficult one, the patient may, intermittently, resort to denial, or partial denial, until his death. Thus he may allude to his end but within a few hours, minutes, or seconds even, he may talk again of a cure.

Why the patient denies, and whether he does so consciously or not are issues which have caused much speculation among terminal care workers (Cramond, 1970; Abrams, 1971; Heusinkveld, 1972; Weisman, 1972a). The patient may deny his impending death for his own comfort, to 'protect' those around him, or because significant others in the patient's environment deny for him and indicate that they expect him to 'control himself' by not mentioning death. The patient soon realises that if those who are important to him are to maintain contact with him during this period, he must behave as he is expected to do. Therefore, if they cannot tolerate any mention of dying, he must not mention it. Accordingly, patients are sensitively selective in choosing different caregivers with whom to discuss matters concerning their illness. Either way, as a *temporary/transient* reaction, denial may be considered helpful in the terminal situation. If, however, the patient maintains this defence throughout the terminal period and makes no attempt to move towards acceptance, it offers an ineffectual way of coping with the situation. Such a patient needs aid in order to advance in his death work.

Denial may be manifest in remarks such as:

It's just one of those things.*

When I go home next week . . .

I'm going on holiday next year.

I'm getting better.

I'm feeling fine.

It's not too bad.

I hope to be back at work by –

The pneumonia is worse than the cancer.

This emphysema is the cause of my trouble.

* It should be noted that statements presented out of context like this may be interpreted in various ways. The underlying emotion is observable, in context, with the aid of each patient's tone of voice and the facial expressions which accompany it.

THE SECOND RESPONSE: ISOLATION

Kübler-Ross discusses isolation together with denial. I shall, however, discuss it as a separate emotional stage in the terminal adjustment process, as it seems to be an intense response, widespread among dying persons.

Having received and blocked the shock of impending death, the patient seems to need to retreat into himself for a period, in order to mobilise his resources to start coping with the situation. Only then can he begin to let go of his denial and allow some awareness to penetrate. Or the withdrawal may signify, as in other threatening situations, that the patient feels danger and withdraws to protect and defend himself. Hence isolation often follows denial and seems to be closely associated with it. For example, denial is isolating if the patient is denying his situation and those in his environment are not. The patient's own protestations that all is well then prevent others from aiding him in his preparation for death. Or, both parties may collude to deny the reality of the situation, again leaving the patient with a barrier between himself and his environment.

Objectively perceived, the process of preparing for death is a solitary one: the patient may be isolated from his fellow men by pain, unshared knowledge, envy of those who are healthy, fear, uncertainty of the future, his own withdrawal, and the taboos which Western society places on the discussion of, and contact with, death. While the religious patient may find God's presence a comfort during the terminal period, for the majority of patients, dying is a lonely process. In addition to the loneliness inherent in all dying, Weisman (1972) points out that many caregivers isolate the dying patient still further on account of their own fears and feelings concerning dying and death. They are uncertain as to how to react to terminal situations. The sense of impotence, helplessness and, at times, despair involved in terminal work renders confrontation with a dying patient intolerable. Consequently, contact with the patient is minimised or avoided altogether.

Isolation may thus be imposed both from inside and outside the patient, by his own denial, by the nature of his situation and by his caregiver's fears concerning dying. Such loneliness is so intense that many writers maintain that the dying patient often finds it more difficult to tolerate his isolation than death itself (Abrams, 1966, and Weisman, 1972).

Isolation may be verbalised as follows:

You don't know how it feels.

You can't know how it feels . . . .

They don't understand.

I don't like to complain, but they can't help me.

I had a vision – I saw myself climbing a mountain on my own, and then – I was all alone on the top, on a grassy plane.

I think I have cancer, but I haven't told anyone.

They don't tell you anything.

I have to manage alone.

I try to work out what's going on.

He came by, but he seemed in too much of a hurry to talk.

I haven't seen the doctor for a week now.

I don't like to bother them; they are all too busy.

No one seems to understand how vital my oxygen supply is.

I try to hide what I'm feeling, so that I don't upset my family.

I don't like to be alone.

I feel like a little pea on the whole ocean.

THIRD RESPONSE: ANGER

Anger is a fairly common feeling experienced by those who face impending death. Once the patient has acknowledged that the threat of death is real, a natural temporary reaction seems to be that of protest and rebellion. Feelings of anger, rage, envy, and resentment predominate. The patient seems to be struggling to answer questions like 'Why?', 'Why me?' and 'Why not him?' The dying person often feels envious of, and therefore resentful towards, those who are healthy. The target of this anger may be the doctor, nurse, team, his relatives, or God.

In this stage the dying person appears to be out of harmony with his fate and his environment. He may display his feelings in aggression, criticism or complaint, all of which signify his discontent. Accordingly this stage is difficult for relatives and caregivers to tolerate. Doctors and nurses are often targets of anger, while relatives are made to feel unwelcome and inept. Their own feelings of grief or guilt may persuade them to avoid further contact with the patient, which only serves to increase his discomfort and anger. The communication underlying such anger seems to me: 'Notice me while I am still alive'; 'I'll soon be gone'; 'Notice my struggle, and help me'; or 'Don't abandon me'. Yet just because of the patient's anger his family may feel uncomfortable in his presence and may therefore avoid contact with him. Thus, hoping to gain attention and avoid abandonment the patient may grumble and complain even more. Such feelings are intensified in the patient for whom independence and control have been lifelong issues, that is, the person who feels vulnerable when he is forced to acknowledge his dependence or to give up his control, and so reacts with rage.

Anger is unhelpful if it entrenches the patient and makes progression beyond this phase more difficult. In particular, used as a long-term defence, anger is unhelpful because it enables the patient to avoid the pain of his situation by focusing on people and things in his external world. In addition, it antagonises caregivers at a time when they are most needed. On the other hand, anger may be useful as a short-lived response during a time of crisis because it mobilises the patient's untapped resources and spurs him to move on in his death work. In practice, anger is seldom neatly distinguishable as long-term or short-term. It may predominate in the terminal crisis; it may reappear from time to time, or it may be completely dispelled, depending upon how it has been understood and responded to by the patient and his caregivers.

Angry feelings may be expressed as:

Why am I being punished?

They don't care.

No one takes any notice.

I asked the doctor what was wrong – and now I'm still waiting to know.

I haven't seen the doctor once since I've been here.

The treatment is doing me no good.

It's not fair.

These people treat you like an idiot. It's my body.

The doctor is no good.

The nurses are lazy.

My relatives are inconsiderate.

The food is awful.

How can there be a God of love?

They only care about the cancer, there's so much else wrong with my life.

Why didn't the doctor tell me so months ago? Now my condition has been neglected.

This treatment won't work. I've had it before.

They make me feel so useless.

What have I done to deserve this?

Why doesn't this happen to the scroungers and layabouts?

THE FOURTH RESPONSE: BARGAINING

While in the bargaining phase the patient begins, conditionally, to accept the fact of his dying. He appears to be saying, 'Yes, it is me, but . . .' or 'Give me a little longer, and then I'll be ready . . .' The contract is often made between the patient and the treatment team, or God, so that there is evidence of the patient's intuitive move along a spiritual dimension. The patient may bargain with his life in exchange for more time, a day without pain, an opportunity to put something right, complete a task, repent, or to achieve one last wish. Such promises may not be kept; or, as in Mrs D's case (case illustration 5), the contract may be faithfully honoured on both sides. This stage is usually less exacting for the caregivers to manage than other stages of adjustment to dying.

Bargains are evident from the following words:

If only I can be at home for Christmas, I won't mind dying after that.

If only I could be sure that I would not suffer asphyxiation, I'd not mind.

If I could go to heaven, it would be worth all this.

I'll go at God's will, but I have much work to do for Him first.

If I could see my son through university, I'd not mind so much.

If only I could get back to the job for a while.

If only I can take my family on one more holiday before I go.

I would sell my soul to have my health back.

I just want to be home to celebrate my daughter's twenty-first birthday, and then you can start treatment.

THE FIFTH RESPONSE: DEPRESSION

Depression is the last stage through which most patients pass before reaching an acceptance of their death. Once the patient can no longer deny his illness his disbelief, rage and bargaining are replaced by a sense of loss, with which depression is usually associated.

There is much to be lost in dying: physical strength, independence, physical attractiveness, identity, usefulness, status, (for some) a limb or part of the body, control, a sense of worth, relationships with loved ones, familiarity with a way of life, and life itself. This state is one of preparatory depression, and may be distinguished from a reactive depression, which contains elements of guilt, shame or aggression turned inward. Preparatory depression may also be distinguished from the depression of mourning which occurs in response to past loss. This depression manifests itself as a silent condition in which there is little or no need for words. The patient may ask for a prayer, or to have something read to him. He may already be occupying his thoughts with things ahead, rather than things past. During this time interference from visitors or caregivers who try, inappropriately, to cheer him up may hinder his emotional preparations for death.

Sadness or depression of this kind appears to be necessary and beneficial if the patient is to die in a state of acceptance and peace. Only those persons who have been able to work through some of their anxieties and depression seem able to reach the final stage of adjustment to dying. This definitive statement is made with the account of Jesus in the Garden of Gethsemane in mind. The reader is reminded that he experienced such anguish that he sweated blood (haemohydrosis), before he reached acceptance ('Thy Will be done . . .') and could endure the rest of his ordeal with dignity. Thus in the terminal situation as in others involving loss, depression appears to be a constructive, if painful, emotion, as it keeps the person in touch with reality. It is likely to reappear from time to time as different aspects of the patient's loss are perceived. It may well exist in silence together with acceptance just prior to death.

Depression may be communicated in the following terms :

It doesn't help to complain.

I feel miserable.

I feel depressed

Not long now.

I'm feeling sad.

I'm desperate enough to try anything now.

I feel as if I have one foot in the grave and the other on a banana peel.

What chance have I got?

It doesn't matter.

It's hopeless – this cancer is the end of everything.

Life is tough.

What's the use?

I've had enough.

It's God's permissible will.

I'm so useless now.

I feel blue.

I feel so listless.

When will it be?

I'm not getting better.

I feel low.

I'm good for nothing any more.

CULMINATING RESPONSE: ACCEPTANCE

The final stage of adjustment to dying is one without despair. The reality of the terminal situation has been faced, raged over, bargained with, mourned and, finally, accepted. It is an experience of completion, achievement or preparedness for what lies beyond. It is a state of calm self-containment. The patient's thoughts are concerned with the future rather than the past, so that loved ones must inevitably be excluded from them. The patient's self-image, far from being destroyed, has been synthesised and integrated and there is a sense of dignity perceptible to both the dying person and those who tend him.

Acceptance is not happiness, but a preparedness to die. It therefore embodies a gradual detachment from former ties to which, until then, the patient has clung. Now he seems willing, and able, to move on. Decathexis has also been noted in the final stage of adjustment to death, so that the patient emerges emotion-free, in readiness to die. Acceptance of imminent death may be expressed in simple words, a smile, silence, planning for events beyond the death, concern for those who remain behind, or an expression of gratitude. Few needs are expressed, although the companionship of a loved one is often requested. Once the patient is assured that he will not be abandoned while he waits, he seems to be saying, 'I am ready', 'I am no longer afraid', or 'Let me go'. His pace of functioning is much reduced; he needs much physical caring, almost like an infant. He may require fewer visitors and analgesics. He may wish to bid most family members farewell, and then to have limited but continued human company while he waits to die. Not infrequently acceptance is characterised by some spiritual preparation for death. For example, the patient's diminished verbal communications may be limited to a request to have a passage from the Bible read to him. Acceptance may be perceived in the following statements.

I'm dying.

Death will be a relief.

Thank you for all you've done.

I can see things in a different light now: I'm quite happy to lie here quietly. Time passes more quickly now. I'd never have had the patience to lie and do nothing before. Now I'm happy to see my lovely flowers, or feel the sun on my face – which I've never thought about before.

I'm not leaving you much, but I am leaving you my love, as your heritage. May that give you courage [said to a daughter].

Acceptance may also be evident in the movement from one statement to another, for example, from 'It could be worse' (that is, 'this is not unbearable') to 'It's no use complaining' (that is, anger) to 'I don't complain because it only makes it worse for everyone if I do' (that is, acceptance which communicates that the patient can contain his feelings; or that he does not wish to complain). Or acceptance may also be evident, where verbal communication is no longer possible, in actions and gestures. For example: a dying person may be concerned that his caregiver has a chair and is comfortable while visiting him. Similarly, a smile, calmness, an uncomplaining manner, patience despite long hospital delays, or dying 'without troubling anybody' in the process may all be expressions of acceptance of the situation.

In some cases acceptance may be communicated in writing, as the following illustration shows:

Case illustration 1: a terminal patient demonstrates acceptance of impending death

MRS E, A 65-YEAR-OLD WOMAN, POORLY EDUCATED, RETIRED, WITH NO CHILDREN, WROTE THE FOLLOWING LETTER FOR HER HUSBAND THREE WEEKS BEFORE SHE DIED. IT WAS FOUND BY HIM AFTER HER DEATH.*

* Permission has been obtained from this patient's husband to print this document; names and identifying details have been deleted.

To my Dearest and Beloved Husband, S——,
I want my funeral service with me taken to our little church, the Methodist where we were married in H—— Street, M—— [suburb], then cremated and my ashes buried in my 'Mother's' grave at P—— Cemetry [sic], after a little service for all my Beloved family, and don't forget I pray for you all and Love you all for ever and ever.
Please all be very very kind to my 'Beloved S' he will be very lost and lonely, so please all of you love him, look after him, and see he has your company often.
God is Good and in the by and by we will all meet once again in the presence of 'God', all will be united and Happy once again.
Your beloved,
J.

Acceptance of death is evident in Mrs E's letter which displays her certainty that death is at hand and her ability to share this fact with others. It shows concern only for those who will remain behind, as is evidenced in her request for a church service for her family, not herself. It conveys Mrs E's certainty that she will continue to live in spirit and will eventually be reunited with her loved ones. The letter demonstrates sad awareness that she will no longer be able to care for her husband (preparatory depression), balanced by contentment that other relatives will be at hand to provide companionship in her place. Finally, Mrs E's letter shows a calm readiness to journey on.

A final point to emphasise concerning the patient's progression through this sequence of emotional stages is that by the time he reaches acceptance he knows that he is dying, whether he has been told or not. Indeed several studies have concluded that by the time most people die they know they are dying and are usually ready (Hutchnecker, 1959).

We have so far discussed six emotional stages involved in coming to an acceptance of the terminal situation: denial, isolation, anger, bargaining, depression and acceptance. Now let us look at approaching death in terms of the tasks that the dying person needs to complete.

Chapter 3

———◆———

SIX TASKS PREPARATORY TO DYING

Continuing our attempt to understand the complicated elements of the terminal crisis we may ask, what provokes the intense feelings described in the previous chapter? I suggest that those feelings occur in response to the activity in which the patient is engaged as he progresses towards an acceptance of death.

My approach is to describe the dying person's work as a set of problem-solving tasks which require his attention. These six tasks are outlined here as though they are discrete and self-contained. In practice, however, the distinctions are not so clear and each task shades into another. The dying person's tasks are:

1 to become aware of impending death;
2 to balance hope and fear throughout the crisis;
3 to take an active decision to reverse physical survival processes in order to die;
4 to relinquish responsibility and independence;
5 to separate the self from former experiences;
6 to prepare the soul for death.

'Achievement' in dying does not necessitate work on all six tasks. Each patient will have work to do in different areas, depending on which of these issues have proved crucial in living.

The terminal crisis is a complicated one, which man does not yet fully comprehend. Consequently, this account is somewhat oversimplified. For example, there is a degree of uncertainty in every terminal situation; the unexpected (that is, a miracle) has sometimes been observed. Pain, physical debility and medical technology may all interfere with the patient's dying work. Denial, projection, fear and subjectivity abound wherever dying or death occurs. In addition, lay and professional caregivers in the environment may collude – consciously or unconsciously – to block the patient's work by confusing and contradicting his growing realisation that he is, in fact, dying (Glaser and Strauss,

1966). These dynamics should be borne in mind in relation to the description of the crisis presented here.

1 AWARENESS OF IMPENDING DEATH

Although the whole of life may be viewed as an opportunity to equip oneself for death, one can only begin to prepare for it after becoming aware that it is approaching. This fact may become apparent at any stage of life but, for some, it arises consciously only once the process of dying actually commences. Thus with whichever issue the patient initiates his terminal crisis work, it appears to be linked with that of coming to realise that he *is* dying.

The patient's work of becoming aware that death is approaching is complicated by several factors. First, it requires a response from him at both thinking and feeling levels. Kübler-Ross (1970a) has observed that, like all awareness processes, this one does not involve an exercise of mere intellectual calculation; if the patient is to tolerate the new knowledge, emotional readiness to confront the terminal situation has to accompany the mental discovery. In other words, this task may be complicated by the uncertainty surrounding whether the person really wants to know that he is dying. Knowing is often accompanied by implications and responsibilities for which he may feel unready. On the other hand, the man who has faced other life-crises with maturity, who has been able to take something positive out of other situations of loss, or who has a firm belief in life after death, *is* likely to want to know that he is dying.

Becoming aware is further complicated by environmental events which are beyond the patient's control. For example, as Kalish (1970) points out, several clues are offered to the discerning patient: the doctor comes less often and talks to him less; his bed may be moved to another part of the room or ward; he looks different; long lost relatives visit, and so on. At the same time, many environmental pressures thwart his acknowledgement of the fact that he has assumed the role of the dying person: for example, he is told that he is looking better, or that he is improving. Another dynamic beyond the patient's control is the quality and quantity of communication offered to him concerning his condition. Whether he is told or not, what is said, when, how and by whom will all affect what and how much of this information he hears, comprehends and can absorb. Hence the patient may be cared for in one of four awareness contexts (Glaser and Strauss, 1966), or a conspiracy of silence may surround his struggle to define himself as a dying person. Either way, the patient often seems able to overcome these complications and comes to know that he is dying, whether he has been told or not.

A fourth factor which complicates the patient's task of becoming aware of his impending death is a lack of certain facts. A degree of uncertainty exists in every terminal situation. The medical diagnosis of 'terminal illness' may be premature or inaccurate. There is thus often some room in every terminal situation for manoeuvre, hope, experimentation, drastic treatment, last resorts, heroic procedures, decisions, resignation and acceptance. Then awareness may take several forms. For example, it may consist of acknowledging that death *may* be at hand (which possibility then becomes certain knowledge only once acceptance is achieved). Or, it may take the form of a suspicion or realisation that death is approaching, accompanied either by an inability ever to verbalise this knowledge openly, or by limited or, sometimes, open discussion of it.

Awareness of dying is, however, seldom consistently maintained over an extended period (Kübler-Ross, 1970a). As with other emotional awareness, the patient is capable of tolerating differing degrees of revelation at different times. Thus a patient may one minute appear to know that he is dying, but behave, a few minutes later, as though he believes that he will recover again. This practice is nevertheless healthy and normal as it brings the patient a little nearer to full awareness with each expression of its dawning.

Case illustration 2: inconsistent awareness of dying

Mrs F, a divorcee of 58 years with carcinoma of the lung, was told by the consultant surgeon in response to her determined questioning that she had a malignant growth in her lung, and that a 'gland' had been removed.

The next day when the social worker visited, Mrs F told her aggressively that all she wanted to know was what was wrong with her and where she stood. She told the social worker that the surgeon had said that there was a growth. She had asked whether it was malignant, and he had said that 'they always were'. 'So now,' said Mrs F, challengingly, 'I still want to know whether mine is malignant . . .'

This example shows the struggle that is involved in becoming aware of, and remaining in touch with an uncomfortable situation: dying. It also highlights one of the many forms which awareness may take. Whether unresolved awareness issues will inhibit parallel work on other tasks or not is, to date, uncertain. As I have indicated at the beginning of this discussion, I think that they would. The person whose habitual life pattern has been one of denial, withdrawal or avoidance will experience difficulty in regard to awareness of dying, as will the person who is frightened of death.

2   HOPE AND FEAR

Throughout the terminal crisis both hope and fear prevail – sometimes at a conscious and sometimes at an unconscious level (Kübler-Ross 1970a). The patient's problem-solving task thus lies in balancing these two emotions. As stated in the extensive literature, fear of dying often reflects a fear surrounding some aspect of living (Rosenthal, 1957 and 1963; Cappon, 1961; Wahl, 1966; Carlozzi, 1968; Le Shan, 1969). In addition, the dying person has much to fear in approaching death: pain and suffering, disfigurement, abandonment, uncertainty, helplessness, loss, deprivation, impending judgement and death itself. Fear may however be balanced by hope (Kübler-Ross, 1972). The two emotions fluctuate according to the state of dying work in which the patient is engaged. At times they may be diminished or modified. For example, once acceptance has been reached, the patient may be more anxious about his family's well-being than about his own. Such fearless dying is relatively rare and is possible only if hope is allowed to balance each emerging fear.

Agreement exists that the patient should never be left without hope. Consequently, caregivers need to understand the content and purpose of hoping in their terminal situation. Hope provides the situation with some meaning from which the patient may gain strength to persevere in the face of fear. For example, the patient may hope, as appropriate, that he will be spared undue suffering, that he will not be isolated in his dying, that he will be adequately cared for, that his efforts will be rewarded, that life after death is a reality, that he will, eventually, be reunited with his loved ones and that his family will manage without him. He may also hope, very often inappropriately, to be cured. However, where medical uncertainty prevails hope of recovery may be appropriate and may, paradoxically, keep despair at bay sufficiently to enable the patient to concentrate on other aspects of his dying work.

Where hope is absent, fear may reign. If the suffering is experienced as meaningless, feelings of hopelessness or despair may set in. All these emotions need to be recognised and worked with if death is to be achieved with dignity. For example, despair may result from the recognition that no man can alter the terminal situation, while hope may lie in coming to acknowledge that God can equip one to cope with it. Table 3.1 shows how hope and fear may affect the terminal crisis by fluctuating, coexisting or recurring in each stage of adjustment. It suggests that what is hoped for or feared changes with each stage of the illness and its accompanying emotional state.

Case illustration 3: fluctuating hope

Fluctuating hope is demonstrated by Mrs I, a 41-year-old wife and mother with disseminated carcinoma, who hoped at first to get better: 'I still have

Table 3.1 Showing how Fear and Hope are modified as they accompany each Psychosocial Stage of Dying Work

Emotional stages of dying work as formulated by Kübler-Ross	Fear: a negative emotion which persists throughout dying work	Hope: a positive emotion which persists throughout dying work
1 DENIAL: the patient denies that he is dying.	The patient fears that he is dying and is afraid of the pain and of death itself.	The patient hopes that he will be cured, and that he will not suffer too much.
ISOLATION: the patient's plight is denied; thus he feels isolated in his terminal struggle.	The patient fears that he will be rejected and abandoned in his suffering. He fears that no one else has ever suffered as he, and that no one understands what he is suffering. Consequently, he fears the unknown.	The patient hopes that human contact will be maintained with him. He hopes that others have mastered this situation; if so, he may do so too, and the way may not be too unfamiliar after all.
2 ANGER: the patient feels angry about his fate.	The patient may fear the wrath of God and the dependence and helplessness of his situation. He also fears that he will appear to be deserting those who depend on him, and feels guilty about this possibility in a protesting way (for example, 'It's not my fault').	The patient hopes that he will be permitted some control over his situation, but that no heavy responsibilities will be demanded of him while he is so dependent and helpless. He also hopes, that his struggle will be recognised and that his family will, somehow, be looked after.
3 BARGAINING: the patient bargains for more time and less suffering.	The patient fears that his bargain will not be agreed upon, and that he will not be able to manage all that he has planned in the time still available to him. The patient who fears judgement may bargain for more preparation time. The patient who fears death may bargain, with his soul, for restored physical health.	The patient hopes that the bargain will hold, that he will be granted a little more time to live and that he will not die –yet. He may also hope that he will be mercifully judged and that he will pass the test.
4 DEPRESSION: the patient experiences preparatory grief and depression.	The patient fears separation and loss of limb, function, role, relationships, identity and life itself. He again fears abandonment, isolation, loneliness and meaningless suffering. He is frightened by his feelings of regret about his past. He fears that his helplessness might make him a burden to others. He fears that he may have suffered in vain.	The patient hopes that he will not be altogether abandoned before he dies; that the separation from loved ones and loss of familiar things will be bearable; and that he will be courageous in bearing his experience. He may hope to be eventually reunited with his relatives. He hopes that the purpose inherent in his suffering has been fulfilled.
5 ACCEPTANCE: the patient accepts that he is dying and prepares to depart.	The patient fears that his relinquishing of control may be perceived as 'giving in'. He fears a loss of dignity, since letting go of life may require that he lets go of his dignity too. He fears that his family may not yet be ready for him to depart.	The patient hopes that his struggle will have been understood and that he will be able to maintain his dignity. Again, he may hope to be reunited with his family in eternity. In the meantime he hopes that his family will be able to manage without him once he has gone.

much work to do . . .'; then to go home just once more to complete her tasks as mother: 'There are many things I want to tell my [adolescent] daughter, things that she should hear from her mother'; then to be allowed to retain her position in the ward:' at least I can face the wall when I am sad, so that no one else can see'; and then that her family would be looked after: 'but don't upset them when you speak to them . . .'

This task of balancing hope and fear is likely to present difficulties to the person whose fears pervade the situation, and to the unbelieving, despairing, hopeless person.

3 AN ACTIVE DECISION TO REVERSE PHYSICAL SURVIVAL PROCESSES

The ability to die appears to require some volition on the part of the patient. Thus when facing impending death the dying person may react consciously; if he is heavily sedated this decision or action may be obviated. Where a reaction is forthcoming it forms a third problem-solving task for the terminal patient. On this point, Weisman and Kastenbaum (1968) stress that acceptance of dying constitutes a positive act and not mere capitulation. Paradoxically, it involves an active cessation of former patterns of control (Weisman, 1972a). Similarly, Saunders (1966a) points out that the act of dying requires more than mere resignation. It is the very opposite of doing nothing. Rayner (1971) supports this view of dying work thus:

> Then perhaps a day or so before the end, the patient seems to give up interest and lets death take him. Many people lapse into uncon-sciousness; others may remain aware, but simply withdraw; a subtle change takes place so that those around usually recognise that death is very close. (p. 237)

Kübler-Ross (1970a) endorses this. See, for example, her description of the reversal process and the struggle preceding it:

> There are a few patients who fight [right] to the end . . . The day they stop fighting, the fight is over. The harder they struggle to avoid inevitable death . . . the more difficult it will be for them to reach this final stage of acceptance with peace and dignity. (p. 101)

The struggle appears to surround the will to live, which has been described in terms of man's hopefulness of what life has to offer (Salzberger-Wittenberg, 1970). Once the individual experiences loss – of hope, or any other aspect of his situation – he often wishes to live no longer. In the terminal situation, however, the dying person voluntarily relinquishes his will to live, not only in response to loss, but also in consequence of the conscious reversal of his physical survival processes. Thus in making the decision to stop fighting and 'to let death take him' it appears that the patient is deciding to move with natural innate maturation processes, which, at this stage, lead to death. When he does so, the will to live is challenged, a struggle ensues, and then a reversal process is set in motion. The resolution of the conflict marks the commencement of the patient's work, of moving from an acceptance of the situation to death itself. Consequently growth during the terminal crisis is reversed. It no longer takes place along a physical dimension. Instead, the patient must divert energy newly liberated from the fight for physical survival for use towards accelerated development along emotional and spiritual dimensions. In this sense there may be a quality of ecstasy, expansion and growth, as energy is freed for creative use (Hineman, 1971). Thus many dying persons have used their foreshortened life-span with vitality and joy.

Case illustration 4: a patient chooses to relinquish life

Mr G, 64-years-old, a retired bank-manager, husband and father of three adult children, had had carcinoma of the rectum for eleven years. From the time of the onset of the illness, Mr G was aware of his terminal condition and made realistic preparation for his death. For months preceding his death he was in hospital, sleeping a great deal, in pain and immobile, but conscious and lucid. For two months his condition remained static. This period of waiting confused and distressed him, as he had been prepared to die and could not understand this delay.

A week before he died, without provocation, Mr G said to his wife, 'I have got to decide – do I give up or carry on, or what do I do?' Thereafter he was calmer, appeared to be given over, spoke very little, went into a coma, and died three days later.

This patient offers a striking example of a third problem-solving task of terminal crisis work. The decision-making element of the situation is seldom demonstrated as clearly as in Mr G's case, where reversal lay in his active acknowledgement that he would not recover. Thereafter he permitted physical deterioration to take its course while he concentrated on bringing other aspects of his being to fulfilment.

Whether this physical reversal process causes the dying person to lose his will to live and his fight, or vice versa, is not yet certain. It does however seem likely that this reversal process will be resisted by the person who fears death and by one who does not yet view his death as appropriate, that is, who very much wants to go on living.

4   RELINQUISHING RESPONSIBILITY AND INDEPENDENCE

Another task for the dying person, occurring almost simultaneously with the reversal of the physical survival process, is that of relinquishing responsibility and independence. As the person reverses his will to live he appears to relinquish that which has enabled him to function as a separate, adult entity: autonomy, control responsibility and independence. He thus appears to be engaged in recapturing a childlike dependence and fearlessness (Kübler-Ross, 1970a) – which is not to be confused with excessive dependence in adulthood.

Weisman views this relinquishing process as a transition from autonomous control to 'counter-control', in which the patient yields to the decision-making of (selected) caregivers (Weisman, 1972a). In this sense, dying may be regarded as a letting go in order to merge with something more extensive than the former limits of the ego have permitted. Again, there is a quality of exaltation, liberation and growth in the accomplishment of this relinquishing task, so that dying need not be viewed as a negative or restricting process. Many patients welcome the expansion and release of death and regret resuscitative measures which reinstate their former lives (Osis, 1961). In giving over * the dying person no longer wishes to change the situation. He submits to a force beyond himself. In this sense, yielding control is not giving in, or giving up, which both denote weakness. Instead, the relinquishing described here is a positive experience. The dying person does not feel defeated, but has come to perceive his impending death as appropriate. (Weisman, 1972a).

Case illustration 5: a terminal patient relinquishes her will to live

A 43-year-old wife and mother was desperately ill with disseminated carcinoma. She experienced extreme difficulty in breathing, but fought with determination for several weeks to stay alive until her last ambition, of remaining with her family over Christmas, had been realised. She spent the day quietly at home with her family. Then, content at having achieved her wish, she gave over her struggle for life and died on the following day.

This example shows the patient's struggle for physical survival, and then her active decision to stop the fight. In letting death take her, she gave over her control.

* Giving over is used here to describe the relinquishing process that follows on the decision to let death happen. It is to be distinguished from giving *up*, which term denotes failure, hopelessness and resignation. Instead, giving over may be seen as a positive, courageous act, a setting aside of the ego defences that have characterised a person's life.

Case illustration 6: death work incomplete: an inability to relinquish control

Mr H, 51 years of age, with carcinoma of the lung, had throughout his life fought for control of himself and his situation. While terminally ill he struggled to maintain conscious control over his breathing, and so of his life. For five months he lay medically ready to die but determined not to give over. The medical staff were baffled by Mr H's continuing struggle, until they understood that he was emotionally unready to die as a result of fear of losing control. Eventually, although weak and emaciated, Mr H remained sitting upright and awake for forty-eight hours in order to continue his breathing. Then he keeled over. Even at the end, there was no acceptance. He had not relinquished life; it had been taken from him.

This example reminds us that man is taught some measure of control over his affairs from early childhood. Consequently, relinquishing control constitutes a difficult task in the work of dying. Weisman (1972a) points out that the task is further complicated when society misinterprets this act as one of resignation or failure. The task of relinquishing independence and responsibility is likely to prove difficult for those for whom control and independence have been essential elements of life.

5 SEPARATION OR DISENGAGEMENT

Once the patient has become aware of impending death, has struggled with his fears and hopes and then with relinquishing his control, he needs to withdraw from life in order to die. Hence the fifth problem-solving task of dying work is that of separating the self from life.

In moving from one life-phase to the next the individual has a sense of progression, and of leaving something behind. The same propulsion appears in approaching death. Death can be accepted only once the patient is prepared to leave life behind him and to detach himself from the former, familiar experiences. Thus Kübler-Ross (1970a) writes that death may be contemplated 'with expectation'. Disengagement may be viewed as a process of decreased social involvement. Kübler-Ross conceives of this gradual separation process as 'detachment'. Her work stresses this aspect of acceptance, which is devoid of emotion. The physical struggle is over. The dying person awaits the long-anticipated event, and prepares for it by withdrawing himself from former relationships and emotions. Decathexis, therefore, leads on to an emotion-free readiness to die (Kübler-Ross, 1970a).

Weisman (1972a) points out that once the dying person is engaged in the process of separation he can no longer be expected to bear responsibility or to maintain intense relationships, since he feels a reduced capacity for life and is responding to it appropriately by disengaging himself from it. It is not his intention to rebuff relatives, although this action may be misinterpreted and feelings may be hurt. For some patients, however, disengagement may have the same liberating effect as the reversal and relinquishing tasks have had, that is, one of freeing the self from wordly ties and responsibilities in order to experience something new. This task is likely to be more easily accomplished by the person who believes that he is going to heaven. In contrast, detachment may be a difficult act if he fears that he is going to hell.

Case illustration 7: a patient disengages herself from family responsibilities

Mrs I, a mother, 41 years old with disseminated carcinoma, had formerly expressed concern over deserting her two sickly children. After some weeks of lingering Mrs I began to disengage her concern for her children, as she had come to realise that God could take far better care of them than she could have done. She said that she was happy to entrust them to Him. Having thus been relieved of responsibility, Mrs I seemed to detach herself and died two days later.

Notice the active part Mrs I played in giving over responsibility and separating herself from life.

Case illustration 8: separating the self from life

Mrs J, 62-year-old mother of adult children with advanced malignant disease, wanted to go and felt that those who tended her (loved ones in her family) were holding her back. She asked them not to do anything more for her, and said: 'Leave me . . .' and 'Let me go . . .' Since Mrs J. had detached herself from most human relationships, she refused to be restrained in her 'departure' and therefore greeted visitors with: 'Thank you for coming. Goodbye.' On her last day Mrs J responded to her husband's inquiry with 'Fine, thank you. Leave me . . .'

Notice again the active part Mrs J played in withdrawing from life in order to die. Perhaps it should be mentioned that her disengagement was facilitated by her keen anticipation of going to heaven. Her last words were: 'There is my dear Lord; there He comes already . . . and my Dad . . .'

In contrast, the dying person who fears that he may go to hell, or who has experienced separation anxiety in life, is likely also to find difficulty in this area of dying.

6 SPIRITUAL PREPARATION

Once the dying person becomes aware of his impending death he is likely to ponder on what lies beyond life. Or some aspect of that which lies beyond death may somehow be presented to him by way of preparation. In this vein many patients have reported their experiences of glimpsing another world (Osis, 1961; Moody, 1976), seeing or meeting with a loved one already dead, or, in rare instances, with a biblical character (Acts 7: 55–6; Moody, 1976) and Hinton (1968a) has reported that many patients have been observed to turn, return, or draw closer to God in preparation for death. Consequently, concern and discussions about religious issues are appropriate during this stage of adjustment (Carlozzi, 1968). In some cases, in fact, acceptance of death is synonymous with calm faith or peace (Kübler-Ross, 1970a). (In this sense, the dignity of dying refers to the dignity of an arisen soul.)

A key issue with which the dying person contends is thus a spiritual one. The soul's preparation for death appears to require as much work, involve as much of a struggle and demand as much realistic acknowledgement of the pain of dying as death's emotional adjustment demands. Spiritual preparation may therefore be described as the ultimate terminal problem-solving task. Religion does not obviate the conflicts of the crisis; it should, however, provide the various participants in the situation with the strength to face and resolve them. An explanation of the importance of this terminal task may be that the soul, or ego, senses that it is about to be liberated. Thus energy formerly used for physical survival is now diverted towards enhanced spiritual development. In this sense the decision to reverse survival processes involves man's free will; the giving over and relinquishing tasks constitute acts of trusting or submitting to the will of God; and disengagement involves not only the detachment of the self from life but the separation of the soul from the body. There is thus a constant interweaving of emotional and spiritual work. For the unbelieving patient this task may take the form of evaluating his life experiences in order to reach an integrated whole.

Controversy reigns as to whether patients with or without faith – of any religion – are more likely to reach an acceptance of death. Abrams (1974) responds that religious faith comforts and supports many patients and should be considered in any programme for optimum management, especially in the terminal stage. While many terminal care workers support this point of view, both Hinton (1968a) and Kübler-Ross (1970a) note that religious patients seem to differ little from those without religion. The majority of patients, however, have some form of religious belief, but not enough to relieve them of conflict and fear. These latter patients need help to make the best possible use of the faith they have (Leslie, 1960). Current literature (Pearson, 1954; Player, 1954; MacLaurin, 1959; and Abrams, 1974) and my own experience (1975) confirm that, alongside the contribution of the social worker and the collective care of the treatment team, the religious faith of the dying person – irrespective of denomination – does play a potentially dynamic role in facilitating his resolution of the crisis. Conversely, the absence of religious faith may, among other factors, hinder the terminal patient's progress in his adjustment to dying. Indeed it is my experience that difficulty in this task is likely to affect work in every other aspect of the crisis.

Spiritual preparation is likely to prove difficult for unbelieving patients, those who do not believe in a life after death; those who have faith, but not enough to aid them through this crisis; those who, after a religious upbringing, have rejected God; those who experience guilt in relation to their lives; and those who fear impending judgement, punishment, or hell (Carlozzi, 1968). This does not mean to say that those who do not believe in an existence after death do not also have need of some integration of their life experiences. Their reflective and contemplative work may, however, take the form of a search for meaning in life, or of work on some other related terminal crisis task, for example, disengagement.

A SENSE OF ACHIEVEMENT AND COMPLETION

Dying can be a positive experience. There is no defeat in dignified dying. On the contrary, great fortitude is needed to lay down what has become familiar, and to move calmly into the future.

Although dying is sad and often difficult, for the patient who has completed his dying work and reached acceptance there is a justifiable sense of achievement. In this connection Saunders (1966a) writes that 'A whole life has been gathered together . . . [Here] is the moment of fullest individuality'. She also highlights 'the achievements that people continually make in their dying'. In describing acceptance Weisman (1972a) refers to a sense of completeness. Kübler-Ross uses the phrase 'the monumental task' of reaching the acceptance of death (1970a). All three writers seem to be endorsing my view in communicating a sense of dignity and self-respect in which there is victory over death.

Case illustration 9: a patient's life culminates with achievement in dying

Mr K, 65 years old, a widower with carcinoma of the lung, had lived a hard, deprived life. He had struggled to cope with life's demands and had suffered physical disability, a troubled marriage and then, after a reconciliation, the death of his wife.

Once ill and himself in need of care, Mr K undertook to care for his stepson and grandchildren who had come to live with him. Mr K refused the offer of his sister to have him in her home where she could tend him, as he did not want to be a burden to her and because he was concerned that his pet would be neglected once he left home.

During the seventeen months of his illness, Mr K grew from a helpless, depressed man into a person who, with relatively little social work help, was able to cope with his financial, domestic and medical affairs. He obtained an old age pension, paid off his house and kept house for his stepson and family. Mr K decided on his own terminal care, thinking in terms of the needs of others rather than himself. Throughout the terminal period he remained calm and accepting, experiencing only short periods of depression. Mr K died in his sleep without fuss, attention, or inconvenience to others. In mastering his own terminal situation, Mr K's sense of deprivation appeared to have been dispelled. Herein lay achievement.

INTEGRATING THE ELEMENTS INVOLVED IN THE TERMINAL CRISIS

In some cases these six tasks appear to require attention in sequence. For example, any of this work will appear unnecessary to the patient who really has no awareness of his dying. The separation and relinquishing work can hardly be undertaken before the physical struggle is over. And for many the act of commending the soul to God is the final one. On the other hand, many of these tasks appear to demand simultaneous attention and seem to exist parallel to each other.

Complete resolution of the terminal crisis may require some problem-solving work on all six tasks which have been listed, thus indicating that dying work may require effort in physical, psychological, intellectual, spiritual and/or social spheres of functioning. Few people however appear to do equal battle in all six areas of potential difficulty, although work on some of these issues does appear to be vital to the mastery of the terminal situation. Other tasks may require little or no work. The tasks do appear to be linked and to influence the outcome of each other. For example, spiritual difficulties may provoke denial, fear and resistance to the relinquishing and separation work required in order to reach acceptance. Which issues will require each terminal patient's attention will be determined, by *inter alia*, his physical condition and his patterns of functioning during former life-phases. Thus the way the person has lived will influence the way he dies (Tillich, 1959).

The interplay of the problem-solving tasks that the dying person is engaged in and the feeling responses that the work provokes in him are presented in tabular form for greater clarity. Table 3.2 highlights the complicated nature of the terminal crisis since it shows that the patient may be required to work simultaneously on the resolution of many related issues. Timing may be a complicating factor: the person who gives over too early may continue in as much distress as the patient who holds on for too long (Oppenheimer, 1967). Ultimately, the timing of a man's death is beyond his control but, mercifully, he does appear

Table 3.2 *Psychosocial and Spiritual Tasks which require Problem-solving work during the Terminal Crisis, where Death with Dignity is a Goal*

Psychosocial and spiritual tasks	progressing through five stages of adjustment to death in response to the task at hand	struggling towards awareness of impending death	balancing hope and fear	taking an active decision to reverse former physical survival processes	relinquishing the will to live, responsibility and independence while at the same time controlling self as much as possible	detaching or disengaging of self from life	turning, returning or growing closer to God
Problem-solving work	movement from denial and isolation, through anger, bargaining, and depression toward acceptance	assimilating intellectually perceived and emotionally experienced clues	permitting both emotions expression, then modifying the contents of both emotions according to the stage of psychosocial work in which the patient is engaged	a struggle and then a rechannelling of energy along emotional and spiritual dimensions; at the same time, moving with innate, natural maturation processes towards death	a gradual return to dependence with dignity; not mere resignation, but the cessation of former patterns of control	separating self from human relationships in preparation for death	accelerated growth along a spiritual dimension in preparation for the liberation of the soul

to be given some part in it by his own preparation for it. Thus while any one of these tasks remain unresolved the patient will either linger at the point of death, unready to die (and divine synchronisation sometimes seems to mean allowing extra time when it is needed) or he will not be able to retain his dignity in dying.

Many issues in understanding the nature of the terminal crisis remain unresolved, issues to which present knowledge does not yet appear to have the answer. In this connection, Glaser and Strauss's (1966) words sum up my experience: 'Persons who are present when a death actually occurs are often struck by the remarkably thin line that stretches between life and death.'

NOTE

The greater part of this chapter has been published elsewhere (Poss, 1980).

Chapter 4

DEMANDS ON THE FAMILY

While the dying person is engaged in his preparation for death considerable demands are made on his relatives to adapt to the impending loss. They too appear to have some specific tasks to complete and respond to this work with intense emotion.

From among the many views which exist on the family's management of their situation, Kübler-Ross's (1970a) ideas again present us with a useful guide. She has observed that the relatives also pass through a sequence of stages of adjustment parallel to those which the dying person experiences. Hence we find both parties moving around within the outlined paradigm of adjustment, at times in harmony with each other, at other times in conflicting stages and in need of synchronisation if their crisis work is to be mastered. For example, where the timing of response differs, the patient may be held back by unready relatives, or rejected by relatives who have completed their adjustment work before he dies.

Let us consider how these stages of adjustment apply to the family. At first the relatives are shocked and deny the severity of the situation, hoping that the patient will soon be well again and that no great changes or adaptation will be demanded of them. Then, as the illness develops, they may set up a conspiracy of silence around the fatal nature of the illness. Both the dying person and friends, relatives and neighbours who are unsure as to how to react are likely to withdraw from the family. As awareness dawns that the patient will not recover, anger and rage seem to prevail. Relatives often demand an explanation and find the apparent senselessness of the situation intolerable. Life without that person seems beyond contemplation. Blame abounds – against the medical profession, the hospital, God, sometimes against the patient who has neglected his health and, most difficult to bear, against themselves, who should have ensured earlier treatment or the like. Anger is then used as attack to defend them from feeling the pain of their guilt and, later, to mobilise their resources to cope with the situation.

Bargaining may take the form of requesting or demanding more time in which to complete some special project, have a last fling together, do something dreamed of but long deferred, indulge themselves, make amends, or do some similar reparation work. Again the bargain may be made with God, the doctor, the patient or between relatives themselves. Then depression follows. The illness has been confirmed or prolonged. As recurrences set in the patient requires more care and the impending death can no longer be ignored. The reality of the loss impinges and the family often mourns in anticipation and preparation of the event. Since several of the patient's strengths may no longer be in operation, for example, he no longer fills his former role in the family and his dependability and vitality are absent, the family reacts appropriately to their disappearance by mourning. They are by then experiencing both actual and impending loss. Grief, depression, sadness, fatigue and other somatic symptoms may manifest themselves in all the family members, or particularly in that relative who is bearing the major portion of the whole family's burden.

Finally acceptance dawns and the family feels ready for the patient's departure. They too have moved through the sequence of shock, loneliness, rage, bargaining and sadness in preparation for the loss. Now death may seem appropriate and they would not wish to delay the patient's death, or prolong his suffering any further. There is often a sense of relief at the patient's release and at the completion of their difficult caregiving task. At the same time considerable guilt may stretch into grief work, and beyond, as they question whether they did in fact do all they could for their dying relative. Acceptance here consists neither of happiness nor of despair. It may be composed of a sense of meaning, or some new awareness of purpose to life and death.

The family's progression towards acceptance resembles the dying person's adjustment in several ways. Relatives are also likely to achieve their goal only if they are able to experience the intensity of the emotions which precede it – particularly the anger and depression prior to acceptance. The hopes and fears which impinge on each stage of the patient's adjustment accompany the family's journey towards their acceptance in like manner. By contrast, one emotion that the family is likely to experience more intensely than the patient is that of guilt. It may be present throughout all six stages of adjustment, as the members question whether the fatal illness could have been prevented, whether they could have done anything else in the situation and, later, whether they could have done more, or been kinder or more helpful to the patient. How they cared for this relative may affect their expectations of their own caregivers many years later, when they themselves face death. Another similarity in the adjustment of both the dying person and his family lies in the fact that these strong emotional reactions described so far are also provoked by the psychosocial and spiritual *work* in which they are engaged, as they prepare themselves for a death in the family.

Thus again my approach is to describe the family's activity as a set of linked problem-solving tasks, at least some of which need to be resolved if the crisis is to be mastered. Some are undertaken as the counterpart of the patient's work in that area and some are initiated by the family in their own right. And, as with the dying person's work, some of them are likely to be undertaken at a conscious and some at an unconscious and/or non-verbal level. Since these tasks have been discussed extensively in the literature,* they will merely be listed here. They include:

1 responding to whichever terminal crisis task their dying relative is engaged in, that is, as corollaries or complementary actors in the situation;
2 reviewing their lives together;
3 evaluating their relationships with the dying person and, as a follow-on, reflecting on themselves and their own lives;
4 dealing with unresolved business in the past;
5 completing any unfinished issues;
6 caring for patient in the present;
7 participating in decision regarding life-prolonging procedures for the patient;
8 using their now shortened time together as creatively as possible in the present;
9 balancing their energies and resources between their own adjustment and their care of the patient and between issues of the past, present and future;
10 handling their guilts in relation to the patient's dying and then his death;
11 planning for the future without the patient;
12 making new resolutions about their own lives as a result of their contact with loss and death;
13 reassessing relationships with God in the light of their encounter with death;
14 realigning the disrupted family system after the death;
15 grief work, including experiencing the intense pain of bereavement, emancipating themselves from bondage to the deceased person, readjusting to the environment in which the deceased relative is missing and forming new relationships and patterns of rewarding interaction (Lindemann, 1944).

* N. Pearson, 1954; National Association of Social Workers, 1960; Carlozzi, 1968; Hinton, 1968a; Kalish, 1969; L. Pearson, 1969; Kübler-Ross, 1970a; Schoenberg *et al.*, 1972; Daniel, 1973; Goldberg, 1973; Abrams, 1974; Burton, 1974; Weisberg, 1974.

As with the patient's terminal crisis tasks, few families are likely to engage in all of these. Some of them, however, will need to be tackled if the crisis is to be mastered. They are listed in an order suggesting some sense of sequence of the work, as if the focus were first on past issues, then present and then future ones. In practice, however, many of them are likely to be linked and to require simultaneous attention, resulting in ambivalent and conflicting feelings and reactions.

The family's adjustment work may be complicated by various factors. For example, the dying person's present need of care may demand so much of their attention and so drain their energy and resources that they have little time left to spend on their own adjustment to the situation. These circumstances may be further complicated by the demands of other members of the family, especially siblings if the patient is a child, and by the game-playing that may by now have set in, in an attempt to protect the patient, and themselves, from the pain of the situation. Other complications in the family's adjustment may stem from the already complex patterns of functioning prior to the onset of the terminal illness. For example, intense emotions are often projected within a family on to that person who, unconsciously, offers him- or herself as a willing receptacle (Salzberger-Wittenberg 1970), so that one member of the family may be seen as particularly strong or disturbed as a result of the events in the family. Or a family member may subtly be pressured into holding a great deal of the whole family's depression, so that he/she remains depressed long after the death. Or unresolved grief work, associated with a previous loss, may erupt as uncontrollable hostility or depression in relation to this impending loss.

The family's need to grieve the loss cannot be overemphasised. Where emotions are suppressed children are likely to feel confused and to interpret the control of feelings as a lack of care for the departed one. As for adults, because the impact of bereavement is so powerful and feelings of hostility and rage so unexpected, they may fear for their sanity (Lindemann, 1944). If these issues are not resolved the future mental health of the family may to some extent be endangered.

I have so far presented the terminal crisis in some detail since our full understanding of it will equip us to help the dying person in his resolution of it. In Part Two we will discuss the caregiver's contribution to the situation in the form of the social worker's response.

Part Two

THE ROLE OF THE CAREGIVER

Chapter 5

CARING SKILLS

A PLEA FOR TRAINING

It is not only the dying person who feels uncomfortable with his confrontation with death. Many writers have acknowledged that doctors, nurses, paramedical staff and chaplains all experience feelings of discomfort, helplessness, fear and some temptation to avoid terminal situations (Player, 1954; Quint, 1967; Carlozzi, 1968; Hinton, 1968a; and Weisman, 1972a).

In this regard, Glaser and Strauss (1966) have studied the behaviour and interaction of doctors, nurses, patients and relatives in four awareness contexts in which terminal patients are generally cared for:

(1) *closed awareness*, in which the patient is not aware of his situation but the staff members are aware.
(2) *suspicion awareness*, or a contest for control, in which the patient suspects that his situation is terminal while the staff is aware of it but keeps it from him.
(3) *mutual pretence*, in which context a ritual drama is enacted: both patient and staff are aware of the terminal situation, both parties are aware that the other party knows, but nothing is said openly.
(4) *open awareness*, in which all participants in the situation are aware that the patient is dying and all talk freely in this regard.

Their work highlights the avoidable discomfort for all the participants in the situation aroused by any awareness context other than an open one. Their work also makes it possible to see how the person's capacity to resolve the terminal crisis will be strongly influenced by the extent and quality of communication that significant people in his environment maintain with him during this final life-phase.

How then to respond to the needs of the dying patient, when our own needs and fears interfere, is a question which merits serious attention. It seems obvious, both from the literature and practice, that just as the patient needs help in mastering his terminal crisis, we, the care-givers, also need preparation, in-service training and ongoing support in order to work in close contact with suffering, dying and death. Since the need for training is closely associated with the quality of the service rendered, the mandate to develop and ensure the worker's skill takes on administrative proportions as well. Accountability to society de-mands that the worker perform at her optimum level. But at the same time cost-effectiveness requires that there is some benefit both to the recipient and the provider of the service. Hence the caregiver's need for training opportunities in which to evaluate her patient's progress and her own cannot be overlooked.

This plea for training is not to be viewed as a case for professional-isation. The learners are likely to include some professional colleagues but also, ideally, the friends, neighbours and relatives of the dying person, who, with some guidance concerning how to care for the patient, remain the best people for the task. Training for terminal care, as for many other service activities, involves the learning of know-ledge, attitudes and skills. The knowledge required has been outlined in Part One. But knowledge about terminal care does not automatically lessen the caregiver's apprehension about her work since subjectivity, denial and projection abound in this field. Hence the accumulation of mere facts regarding dying and terminal care is unlikely to constitute adequate preparation for the task. The caregiver needs, instead, to be willing to look at her own self in relation to her work and to invest her-self in continuing adult learning in order to develop her skills in this area. Understanding, insight and knowledge may therefore be viewed as starting points to attaining skill.

The additional preparation that terminal care work requires thus appears to involve the development of skill, either on a course prior to the commencement of the work and/or as in-service training. Ideally, both should be made available to the caregiver, as one valuable com-ponent of ongoing training is the accompanying support it offers to learners. Skill may be developed through supervision, consultation, staff development programmes, case conferences, workshops, ward meetings and/or skills training courses. An outside consultant may be enlisted to act as monitor, to identify difficulties and/or to comment on the processes at work. Whatever form the training takes, it should take both content and process of teaching into account, as the mode of teaching needs to fit the content. The more congruence there is between what is being taught about caring, the use of time and particularly about endings, and the way the teacher demonstrates these precepts in her teaching, the more likely the worker will be to use her learning experience as a model on which to base her interaction with dying patients. The process of learning about terminal care, if appropriately commented upon, may be an ideal way of linking some aspects of the here and now with those aspects of the dying process under discussion. Another issue which training for terminal care should take into account is the attitude with which several caregivers, and social workers in particular, may approach this field of work. There was a time in the development of several caring professions, like social work, when help consisted of enabling people to accept and adjust to inevitable conditions, as is appropriate to dying. Today, however, social work may be the most optimistic and future-oriented of the human service professions, believing that some improvement is possible, no matter what the problem. Since problems are, by definition, phenomena to be battled with and reduced, not facts to be accepted and dealt with as realities of the situation, training needs to cater for these attitudes and the changes in perspective that may be required of the learner.

Changing attitudes and developing skills are not easy activities. The training required for terminal care work thus demands considerable personal involvement and commitment on the part of the learner. The cost of such commitment is high, but in Saunder's (1965, 1966a) view, it needs to be. She has warned caregivers that when close contact with a dying person ceases to be difficult and challenging it may well be time to withdraw from the situation in order to assess what is happening – both to the patient and to herself. For example, while this work is continuously experienced as complicated, those very encounters with difficulty, uncertainty and pain, which yield no apparent results, may be useful to the caregiver in keeping her in touch with some of what her patient is enduring. On the other hand, once work with a dying patient seems easy the caregiver is likely to be colluding, denying or blocking some of the patient's experience.

THE SKILL REQUIRED: AN ABILITY TO TOLERATE CLOSE CONTACT WITH DYING AND DEATH

On the whole the skills required for social work in terminal care are those required in all social work fields. But as a result of observations in the field, clinical consultation and a study of relevant literature, I have become aware of an additional skill which is required specifically for the practice of terminal care work, that is, the ability to tolerate close contact with dying and death. I want here to stress that *all* terminal care workers need to develop this capacity if optimal patient care is to be ensured. For our present purposes, however, this skill will be discussed as it affects the social worker.

Many writers have commented upon the caregiver's own feelings concerning death as constituting a crucial dynamic in the terminal situation. Kübler-Ross (1970a) stresses that unless the worker has come to terms with her own feelings concerning dying and death, she cannot become an effective caregiver to the dying patient. She states that:

It is the persistent nurturing role of the therapist who has dealt with his or her own death complex sufficiently, that helps the patient overcome the anxiety and fear of his impending death. (p. 41)

and

If all of us could make a start by contemplating the possibility of our own personal death, we may effect many things, most important of all the welfare of our patients, our families, and finally perhaps our nation (p. 116)

Kennedy (1960, pp. 23–31), MacLaurin (1959) and Birley (1960), agree that the social worker's unresolved feelings and fears of dying and death are a major cause of avoidance of the terminal situation. Consequently, as has been stated, terminal care remains a relatively neglected area of social work practice (Olsen, 1972). In discussing the terminal care worker's preparation, Weisman (1972a) writes that professional credentials and field of specialisation are less important than the capacity to be there.

That ability 'to be there' may also be described as a tolerance of close proximity with dying and death, which thus constitutes a prerequisite caregiving or social work skill for terminal care work. This competence is required in order to cope with the issues which frequently confront the worker in terminal care: for example, suffering, stress, dependency, hopelessness, despair, suicide, euthanasia, faith or its absence, dying, death and bereavement. Such topics are likely to make demands on the worker at various levels: emotional, intellectual, moral, social, spiritual and practical.

Of what then does this terminal skill consist? I suggest that it involves a combination of several related elements: attitudes, capacities and personal qualities which make it possible for the caregiver to tolerate close contact with dying and death. I believe that while some people may begin terminal care work with this skill, those who do not have it can learn it, if at some cost. It may therefore be useful to identify its various elements as follows: (a) the use of the caregiver's self, her philosophies and feelings; (b) her ability to share in suffering, conflict and anguish in the terminal situation; (c) her own hopes and fears in relation to dying and death; and (d) the role of her religious beliefs in a therapeutic relationship with a dying patient. The outcome of developing this skill of tolerating close contact with death is that the social worker is likely to take a fairly active role in the terminal situation.

The use of the social worker's self, her philosophies and feelings
Traditionally, social work has demanded a skill embracing a

. . . capacity to listen – and to hear, – to be reliably alongside people, to understand what it feels like to be in their situation – and why – and to convey some kind of strength that makes it possible for the other person to begin to cope. (Younghusband, 1973, p. 35)

These words aptly describe one element of the skill of the social worker also in terminal care work. Her own personality, ideas, feelings, values, beliefs and morals, that is, her self must, to some extent, influence her response to frequent, close contact with dying and death and, consequently, her ability to remain in the terminal situation.

Where the social worker's own philosophies, ideas or beliefs are mentioned, the question of imposing these values on to her client is frequently raised, and may lead to accusations in this regard. In reply, Stewart has stated that the worker brings herself, and her values, to each casework relationship.* Whatever the worker's philosophy is it affects her professional relationships to the extent that it enables her temporarily to contain her client's feelings. Thus, what the worker brings to her client is her degree of ability to contain or 'hold' something emotional. In Salzberger-Wittenberg's (1970) terms the social worker's ability to 'hold' the emotions which the patient experiences enables him, eventually, to bear these feelings himself. She cautions the social worker to distinguish her needs from those of her dying patient. For example, in terminal care work where feelings of hopelessness and helplessness may render the situation intolerable to her the social worker frequently experiences a strong temptation to respond to her own need to do something. If she can resist the urge to change the situation, to put things right, or to aim, inappropriately, at a cure for the dying patient, she will be able to receive and hold the feelings which the patient experiences as intolerable. Such use of the social worker's personal philosophies is not an imposition of her values onto a powerless client; it is, however, a dynamic factor in their interrelationship.

The social worker's ability to share in suffering, conflict and anguish in the terminal situation
Another element of tolerating contact with dying involves the worker's capacity to share in suffering, conflict and anguish. For example, in setting treatment goals, the social worker in terminal care may be tempted to aim at the relief of suffering to the extent, at times, of avoiding any confrontation of the real issues at stake. The view of the functional school of social work, of conflict as 'not necessarily dysfunctional' is helpful here. In this sense, Smalley (1970) writes that the

* Seminar discussion on social work in terminal care with social work students, University of the Witwatersrand, Johannesburg, October 1973.

social worker 'facilitates the full experiencing of the conflict which presently exists'.

Applying this concept to terminal care, the social worker enables the patient to experience and tolerate the anguish of the situation in order to come to terms with it and to reach acceptance. This statement is not to be confused with inducing suffering or provoking conflict (for example, by breaking down defences) in order to help the patient adapt to dying. Instead it warns us simply not to block the patient's expression of the full extent of what he is enduring, which is often done because we, the caregivers, cannot bear to be in the presence of such suffering.

Agreeing with this idea, Le Shan (1969) writes that the honesty of the terminal encounter rules out 'kindness'. The task of the social worker in terminal crisis work is to facilitate the patient's conscious experience of what is happening to him. In Smalley's (1970) terms the social worker works with the conviction that a constructive and supported experience of conflict or difficulty can be creative.

The social worker's hopes and fears in relation to dying and death
A third element in which the social worker's self influences the terminal situation relates to her own hopes and fears in relation to dying and death. In order to cope with the fear of death, the social worker needs to view death as a natural life event. She needs to contemplate her own death, acknowledge her fears and, if necessary, she should seek help in dispelling them. Since fear of death reflects a fear of life, the area in which she is likely to work is that of current life conflicts. (Rosenthal, 1957 and 1963).

While the social worker is beset by fears of death, she is likely to convey these feelings to her patients. In similar vein, her hopefulness or lack of hope concerning life, life after death and the help she is offering is also likely to communicate itself to the dying patient. In this sense Rapoport (1970) talks of 'elements of hope and therapeutic enthusiasm' as vital forces in any helping situation. It is important, however, that the worker and the patient both hope realistically and that they do not hope in a denying, colluding or unrealistic way for a cure.

Hope and fear are non-verbally communicated and consequently cannot be hidden or simulated. The worker either feels genuinely hopeful about what can be offered to the patient, or else she communicates fear and/or despair. Hence she needs to come to terms with her own fears and hopes in relation to death in order to tolerate continuing contact with the dying patient.

The role of the social worker's religious beliefs in terminal care work
A final element which influences the social worker's ability to tolerate

terminal care work is the role which her religious beliefs – if she has any – play in the situation. The worker who does not have any spiritual faith may need to examine what effect her own views have on herself and her work with dying patients.

A number of writers have listed the worker's faith as a prerequisite for work with dying and death (Player, 1954; MacLaurin, 1959; Birley, 1960; and Leslie, 1960). Player (1954) discusses it as a determining factor in the worker's attitudes to the dying patient and writes that, 'Maybe we can only approach [this work] with sincerity if we have religious faith ourselves.' MacLaurin (1959) suggests that the value of the social worker's faith lies in her resulting courage and joy, which enable the patient to meet the problems of life with increased strength and confidence. I want to stress, though, that what is communicated to the client, usually non-verbally, is not only her courage or joy (such as it may be) but her hopeful approach to problems, suffering or death; that is, an approach which, although unspoken, carries a conviction that there can be meaning in suffering and in dying, and that it is possible for man to come to accept impending death.

How then does the worker's faith help in terminal care work? I believe that she will be aided if her religious beliefs, irrespective of denomination, serve two purposes:

(1) assure her that there is a supernatural force who is benign and present, so that she is not alone in this difficult situation. For example, from the Judaeo-Christian point of view, faith in almighty God assures the worker that both she and the patient are not mere victims of a malevolent force or of chance, but dignified human beings who are loved and cared for, even in dying, and who are given strength to bear all that is permitted;

(2) make the relationship between life and death clear, give some meaning to life and death, assure her that death is part of life and/or indicate what the state of death is like. For example, belief in life after death means that the struggle involved in dying with dignity may be viewed as a preparation for life in another dimension.

The clearer these views are, the easier it will be for the worker to stay in close contact with dying.

Leslie (1960) observes in this regard that the faith of the helping person is almost inevitably drawn into the terminal situation, since the nature of the crisis is substantively different from other life crises in which this practice would not be permissible. He confirms, however, that the worker is seldom called upon to profess her faith in words; more frequently she is required simply to live her faith, and leave the rest to God. To those social workers who will disagree with the above approach, Player (1954) writes, 'Even if for the social worker herself any organized religion may appear unnecessary, it is only realistic to know that for her client, it may be the most important thing in life'. If, therefore, the social worker feels unable to respond appropriately to the patient's spiritual preparation for death, she should draw his minister of religion into the caregiving team.

ONE OUTCOME OF TERMINAL CARE SKILL: AN ACTIVE SOCIAL WORK ROLE

The worker who has developed skill in maintaining close contact with death will be equipped to take an active role in the terminal situation. Player, among others, confirms that on account of the incapacitating nature of the patient's weakness and the family's bewilderment, the social worker in terminal care should take a fairly active, responsible, initiating and direct role. It is termed 'active' because it recognises that the patient in his yielding state may no longer be able to take responsibility and ask for the care he needs, but instead will at times have to depend on the caregiver to recognise and respond to his needs, unasked. This statement should not be misunderstood. It does not mean that the worker takes an organising or controlling role, or that the terminal patient is placed in a passive infantile position, or that the worker is not aware of the potential persecutory anxieties in the situation. On the contrary, the dying person's active persevering adult efforts need to be facilitated in order that he may master the crisis. The social worker's active role in terminal care work thus consists essentially in responding to the processes already at work within the patient. She enables inherent emotional and spiritual maturation to take maximum effect, chiefly by recognising it, commenting on it and not blocking it when it appears.

The social worker thus responds to what is already happening in the patient's psychosocial and spiritual life. And since Saunders (1966a) has found that the integrity and honesty of his unmasked self prevents his responding to anything but that which is true to himself, the social worker does not need to tell him what to do, induce changes or modify attitudes and feelings. Instead she sometimes puts into words for him those feelings and issues which she senses are filling his head and heart at that time. In doing this she 'holds' the emotions and so conveys reassuring comfort and understanding. Without having spoken more than a few sentences the patient who is too ill to speak much is thus enabled to 'express' his feelings. In verbalizing what the patient is experiencing, the worker is conveying the naturalness and normality of his experience. In this way, fears of madness and despair need not be added to the patient's already considerable realistic fears concerning his terminal experiences.

This role may therefore be aptly described as an active social work role, which constitutes a therapeutic element in the terminal situation. In summary, let me restate that in order to fulfil this active role the worker must possess a clear understanding of the terminal situation and its dynamics, and must have come to terms with those elements of terminal skill which influence her ability to work in close contact with dying, that is, her use of herself, her tolerance of conflict, her hopes and fears and her own religious faith, or alternative philosophy of life.

Case illustration 10: the social worker's ability to tolerate close contact with dying and death

Mr N, a 68-year-old, twice-married divorcee, had had carcinoma of the stomach for one and a half years. During that time he had been treated at the hospital's chemotherapy clinic as an outpatient. Consequently he was known both to staff and patients as a well-groomed active, cheerful and colourful person. He had dabbled in many occupations and had a keen interest in antiques and in old guns. Mr N had received non-intensive social work service approximately every two months. While he responded to the chemotherapy treatment he was relatively well and there was no need to offer him more intensive care.

Mr N frequently used denial as a defence mechanism. For example, he was sure that social work had value in a hospital, but for others, not himself. It seemed important to him to maintain control over his life and situation. Consequently the thought of deteriorating health, dependence, uselessness, or of becoming a nuisance to his family made him apprehensive when considering the future. Denial was also evident in Mr N's approach to his illness. For example, he interpreted his medical history as 'I had an operation a year ago for a non-malignant tumour. But it went wrong, leaving an infected tummy and permanent diarrhoea, for which I have had X-ray treatment. Otherwise, I am OK.'

Ambivalent fear concerning dying was expressed during the first interview, when Mr N said that everyone had to die somehow; he had had a good innings, 68 years, and had enjoyed them all. Later in the same interview, however, he said that he would not want to know if his condition were malignant. If he knew he had six months to live, he would see no purpose in waiting; he would take an overdose (of drugs) that night.

CIRCUMSTANCES OF THE INTERVIEW

After eighteen months of chemotherapy treatment, Mr N was admitted to hospital in the final stages of carcinoma. By that time, after five months of social work contact, he was known as 'a denier', for whom control and independence were important. He fluctuated between a closed awareness context and one of mutual pretence. Although the ward staff had informed the social worker that Mr N was a little confused, she approached him wishing to assess his emotional state without preconception.

INTERVIEW WITH MR N (in hospital)

Aim: to facilitate terminal crisis work; to support Mr N as he entered his final life-phase.

Record	Comment
The worker began the session by discussing the circumstances of Mr N's hospital admission [1]. He denied his most recent symptom, rectal bleeding, but spoke vehemently concerning his diarrhoea: 'It can drive you mad.'	1 In an effort to 'begin where the client is', and 'move at the client's pace', the worker focused on Mr N's medical condition. Questions which motivated the worker's thinking at this point were: what did he perceive to be the problem? How did he feel about it? How much did he know?
In reflecting upon his total situation, Mr N said that the blow of his only son's recent death (two months earlier) was mild in comparison to what he was now experiencing. He felt that he had not deserved this blow of being so helpless and dependent in hospital, where he was treated like a child and an invalid [2].	2 The worker understood that the blow lay in having lost his control, and enabled Mr N to verbalise it and to clarify those elements in his situation which were causing him depression and anxiety. She actually put his helplessness into words for Mr N so that he, in his weakened state, merely had to nod acknowledgement (an example of her active role).
Having acknowledged, in words, feelings which had hitherto been denied, Mr N felt despair at the full extent of his helplessness and loss of control and expressed his inability to tolerate the situation by saying that he wanted to die [3].	3 The worker had purposely enabled Mr N to move towards an open awareness context in which dying could be realistically acknowledged and prepared for. Her own

Record

Comment

comfort in the presence of dying enabled her to stay calmly at Mr N's side while he explored his terminal situation. (This is an example of her use of herself and her philosophy to 'hold' the patient's anxiety – the first element in terminal care skill.)

The worker nodded her understanding of his desperate feeling [4].

4 This was the first time that Mr N had discussed his feelings with another human being. It appeared to the worker that he found his loss of control and status intolerable, and that this loss caused his desperate feeling. He was not yet able to respond to the next stage of his illness, that is, dying itself.

'Can you help me to die?' he asked. The worker said nothing for a while [5] and then asked whether he felt that he was so near to the end. 'I don't feel near the end, but I want to be. Shall I take aspirin or Codis? ... You know but you won't tell me ... '

5 The worker missed the cue Mr N gave to take up his feeling of despair. Instead she focused on his feelings concerning dying.

The worker said 'No', calmly but with firmness [6] Both the worker and patient knew that Mr N was referring to suicide, although the word was not mentioned.

6 Recognising Mr N's despair, the worker chose not to focus verbally on the feeling which was already intolerable to the patient, but intended instead to convey to Mr N that there was no need for panic or a frantic attempt to change the situation in order to regain control. By stating firmly that she would not help him to die, she hoped to contain Mr. N's feelings, rather than discuss them verbally. In this way, she conveyed, non-verbally, *her* feeling that the situation was difficult, but tolerable. She also intended to convey that she would share in it with him, to the end (this is an example of her ability to share in

Record

Mr N asked how much longer he had (to live) [7] and mused that he would never go to the clinic again. The worker remained silent while he contemplated this loss, feeling no need to reassure him, falsely, that he would recover.

Thinking about the clinic, Mr N mentioned the consultant (that is his doctor), saying that he was a good chap. It was a pity that he was married, as he would have been just right for the social worker [8].

Comment

suffering, conflict and anguish, the second element of this terminal care skill).

In saying that she would not help the patient to take his own life, the worker drew on the fourth element of terminal care skill, that of using her religious beliefs in the situation. Her certainty that almighty God was present, benign and able to support both her patient and herself through this difficult period enabled her to withstand the patient's pleas to end it all. This action also demonstrates the worker's use of the third element of terminal care skill: her own hopes and fears in relation to dying. Because she was not afraid of death and felt hopeful about what Mr N might still achieve on earth before he died, about the reward that his suffering might earn him and about the value of the help she was offering him, she felt no need to change Mr N's situation.

7 It seemed that the worker's response had to some extent contained Mr N's feelings since he was then able to speculate upon various aspects of his present situation, rather than wishing only to escape it. In talking of the clinic Mr N was experiencing a natural sense of loss of former activities and independence.

8 The worker understood that, on account of the regression which often accompanies severe illness,

Record

Mr N said that the worker was a nice person; he liked her and had let her talk to him because he had liked her, but he did not like social workers probing into private affairs. He had no special problems [9].

Responding to Mr N's denial, the worker moved with Mr N into safer areas. She inquired into available facilities for his care and asked if she could be of service to him. He told her that a daughter and son-in-law were taking care of practical matters but she could visit him again, and come to his home [10] although he did not know how long he would be in hospital.

Then, Mr N talked angrily about the doctors, saying that he did not believe them, 'they kidded one along'. The worker understood that Mr N was angry at not being in control of his own situation and said so[11].

Comment

Mr N may have been needing to perceive his doctor and the worker as caring mother and father figures. She did not, however, make this transference interpretation.

9 Mr N appeared to be thanking the worker for her acknowledgement of his feelings. But immediately he had acknowledged to himself that he *had* any feelings, an action contrary to his habitual behaviour pattern, he needed to ward the worker off again and keep her at a distance. Consequently he denied that he had any special problems.

10 Mr N was asking, in his denying way, for the worker to continue her relationship and her service to him.

11 Mr N was angry because he was no longer being involved in decisions that were made on his behalf. By recognising these emotions, the worker enabled Mr N to verbalise his feelings concerning his caregivers – another demonstration of her active role.

Record   *Comment*

As if to prove to himself that he was
not dependent on the doctors he
said, 'I've had a good life; I'm ready
to blow my brains out . . .' [12].

12 The cycle of thoughts appeared
again: 'I've been self-sufficient,
now I am no longer in control;
I want to regain control; I
want to take the ultimate decision concerning my life; I don't
want others to take it for me;
but I can't; I'm helpless; this is
intolerable; help me to die.'

Mr N continued: 'and yet when I
look around the ward and see all
these sick people, then my diarrhoea
and discomfort are nothing' [13].

13 Having brought himself again to
his most intolerable feeling of
helplessness, Mr N needed to
deny his plight, by comparing
himself with others.

The worker agreed that that was one
way of viewing the situation and
suggested that they should discuss it
again when next she visited]14[.

14 Since this comparison left Mr N
with his habitual defence pattern
intact, the worker felt it appropriate to terminate the interview.

ASSESSMENT

Mr N had made progress in being able, if only temporarily, to acknowledge
his feelings concerning his terminal situation. There was evidence of his
fluctuating ability to acknowledge the fact of his impending death. Various
stages of adjustment to dying were evident: denial, isolation, anger and depression. Problem areas included reversing physical survival processes and
relinquishing control.

FURTHER PLANS

Mr N should now be seen more intensively than during the past five months.
Continue to facilitate his terminal crisis work: focus on Mr N's despair
concerning his loss of control over his life.

Mr N was seen by the social worker four times more in the two weeks
before he died.

This illustration demonstrates all the elements of terminal care skill
which we have discussed so far, that is, the worker's ability to be in

close proximity with dying and death, and a fairly active social work role in terminal care. The worker's active role was evident in her putting Mr N's thoughts and feelings into words for him without specifically being asked for help. In recognising the plea behind his behaviour and responding to it, unasked, she was meeting a need that is frequently met only in a relationship of intimacy or dependence. Hence the description of this role as 'active'. What the worker offered to Mr N was her unafraid ability to remain with him and to contain his feelings at a time when other professional and family caregivers were avoiding and deserting him – an example of the use of the first element in terminal care skill, that of using her self, her feeling and philosophy to hold anxiety and to avoid the temptation to *do* something to make the patient's situation bearable.

The illustration also shows the social worker's response to an issue with moral and spiritual overtones: the patient's wish to take control of the situation by committing suicide. The worker did not need to take a stand on his decision, since he did not ask for her opinion. He did, however, invite her assistance, which she refused firmly, at the same time recognising the despair which prompted his request. The worker's refusal to assist Mr N to take his life drew on her own religious standards. Stewart (1970) states that this kind of use of the worker's own values constitute an acknowledgement of the difference between herself and her client and an acknowledgement of the client as an adult person who is free to reject the worker's ideas.

Chapter 6

———◆———

CARING FOR THE DYING PERSON AND
HIS RELATIVES

Once we understand what the dying person is experiencing and something of our own reactions to the situation, we can begin to help him to master his crisis. Although this book is intended for many caregivers, a social work perspective remains in focus. But I want to stress that the adoption of a social work standpoint is not intended to imply that the social worker is best equipped to respond. Most of the caring and service to be described in Part Two may be carried out by any member of the team. The capacity to do this work is what is important, rather than the profession of origin.

The caregiver's efforts to aid the dying person in the resolution of his crisis may be viewed as a response to the patient's own work. The social worker's response may take the form of work with the patient or his family directly, or work with colleagues in the situation on the patient's behalf. This chapter deals with direct or clinical work – undertaken individually and in groups with the patient and his family. It includes three social work functions: terminal crisis work, both with the dying person and his relatives, social group work and environmental management.

TERMINAL CRISIS WORK WITH THE DYING PERSON

The term 'terminal crisis work' is used from two points of view: that of the patient and that of the caregiver. First, as defined in Part One, it describes the patient's efforts to resolve his terminal crisis. At the same time, it is used to signify those caregiving interventions which aim to aid him and his family in the resolution of their terminal situations and so to facilitate dying with dignity. In other words, from the social worker's point of view terminal crisis work refers to the counselling aspects of the service, which constitute her response to the dying person's crisis work. Its content involves counselling in various areas of the terminal crisis, as we have discussed in Part One. In other words, the area of the patient and family's struggle needs to be identified; the cause of the difficulty is assessed; and work can then begin in that area of dying – usually by focusing on that area of living. Terminal crisis work embodies many principles and practices of medical social work and draws particularly upon the theoretical perspective of 'crisis intervention' (Rapoport, 1965 and 1970). It may be undertaken with the dying person and/or his family, individually and/or in a group.

One prerequisite in terminal crisis work, characteristic of all counselling and psychotherapy, is that of engaging the adult part of the patient's functioning in order to work with him on holding and responding to his own childlike needs. This point is stressed because two dynamics may militate against it and tempt us to infantilise the dying person: the medical model often unconsciously provokes the patient's child-self and loses sight of the adult; and at the same time the yielding process of dying enables some early needs – for example, dependence – to re-emerge and exist undefended just prior to death.

Case illustration 11: terminal crisis work in an initial interview with a patient

At the time of first contact with the social worker, Mrs D, 41 years old, with carcinoma of the breast and the lung, had been attending the chemotherapy clinic for four months.

CIRCUMSTANCES OF REFERRAL

Although Mrs D's prognosis was estimated at three to four years, she was referred to the worker by one of the clinic attendants with the comment that, 'She is such a nice person, she'll be one for your work. She waited fifteen years for a child, and now that she has a little boy, she's got cancer.'

INITIAL INTERVIEW (at the chemotherapy (outpatient) clinic)

Aim: to establish contact with Mrs D; to assess her situation with a view to offering intensive or non-intensive social work help; to set a contract accordingly; to initiate terminal crisis work.

Record	*Comment*
The social worker introduced herself, the social work service and the research project.	
Then in response to questioning Mrs D told the worker that she had begun to feel ill three years ago. Six months later carcinoma of the breast had been diagnosed and she had undergone a mastectomy. Since that time she had known that she had	

Record

cancer. She said that she had 'felt nothing' [1] on being told the diagnosis. At first she couldn't believe it [2] 'It is such a terrible word; it means I'm dying.' The worker nodded, acceptingly, said how hard it must be to know that and asked whether she would have preferred not to have been told [3]. Mrs D said not, and then said, adamantly, 'People should be told; I know there are a lot of patients sitting out there (in the clinic waiting area) who don't know what they've got. They should be told. How else can they do the things they want to do?' The worker asked Mrs D what things she still wanted to do and she replied, 'I want to see my son through school, and university, and married, and us retired and living and growing old gracefully' [4].

Again the worker nodded acceptance, without taking up the contradiction of Mrs D's feelings. Instead she focused again on the medical details [5]. Mrs D told the worker that a year after the mastectomy, she had had an ovarian oblation.* Since her fortnightly attendance at the chemotherapy clinic she had been well for one week, while each alternate week in which she attended the clinic had to be discounted, as the injection made her very ill. Consequently, she had to do two weeks' cooking and housekeeping in the week in which she was well.

The worker helped Mrs D to verbalise what this way of life meant to her: it was a constant reminder that she was ill; it was a nuisance; Mrs D felt useless during her 'off'

Comment

1 and 2 The worker noted the reactions of shock and denial.

3 The worker did not confirm or deny Mrs D's awareness but acknowledged the feeling underlying her statement.

4 The worker noted Mrs D's ambivalent and temporary awareness of impending death.

5 The social worker did not confront the patient with her contradiction in feeling or thinking. To do so would have been threatening, and might have broken through a defence of which she had need. Thus the social worker noted the threat as an area of possible future work, and moved back into safer areas of Mrs D's situation.

* Surgery to render the ovaries inactive, on the assumption that the control of the hormonal environment of a tumour may retard its growth.

CARING FOR DYING PERSONS AND RELATIVES 61

Record

weeks; and she dreaded her fortnightly visit to the clinic, the pain of the injection, and the unpleasantness of its after-effects.

Concerning her family, Mrs D told the worker that her husband was a building inspector, somewhat older than herself. They had been married for twenty-one years and Mrs D felt that it was a good marriage. Her son was 6 years old. They had waited fifteen years before they could have a child. The worker commented that Mrs D might feel sad at the thought of being so ill while her son was so young [6]. She agreed, but said that she could see a purpose in the situation in that her husband would still have a companion once she died; he would have some one they both loved. In this God had been good. Mrs D described herself as a person who loved things that were clean and open, like flowers and nature. In herself and her home she was clean and methodical. At times she was stubborn and impatient about having things done her way. She did not regard herself as loving, warm or affectionate, although she did love her family and would do anything for those she loved. She said she was not demonstrative in her feelings [7].

In discussing her faith, Mrs D cried as she said that God had been so unfair to them. The worker clarified that she was feeling angry. She responded vehemently, 'Yes, angry is the exact word. I'm very angry about

Comment

6 The worker linked Mrs D's feelings with her earlier display of awareness of dying. In so doing, the worker demonstrated her willingness and ability to tolerate the thought of dying, thereby freeing Mrs D to follow suit, if she should wish to do so. At the same time, however, the words used allowed Mrs D to evade the harshness of her situation, if she needed to do so.

7 The worker noted: clean, methodical, stubborn, impatient to have things done her way and undemonstrative. A pattern of rigidity and control suggested itself. The worker also noted Mrs D's strength in being able to appraise herself.

Record

it. It's so unfair. I've been good, honest, clean, open and uncluttered all my life. Why don't the dropouts and the drunks get this?' The worker agreed that it must seem unfair at times and that the injustice of the situation was difficult to accept. Perhaps there was no temporal justice, but there was eternal justice . . . she asked whether Mrs D believed in an after-life [8]. Mrs D said not, because if there were, a friend's husband, who was very close to his wife, would have come back to her.

Mrs D asked whether the social worker believed in an after-life. The worker replied that she did, and said that she believed that although Mrs D's present situation made so little sense to her, she felt sure that there was a purpose in it and that perhaps it would become clearer to Mrs D in time [9].

The worker asked Mrs D what helped her when she was feeling sad [10]. She said that when she was depressed she cried. If her husband was there, he gave her a cup of tea

Comment

8 The social worker introduced religious issues in order to assess the total situation and possible resources in it.

9 The social worker answered the patient's question honestly and then reflected it back to Mrs D's feeling of anger and meaninglessness. She hoped, thereby, to indicate to the patient that it was permissible to express angry feelings if she wished to do so. At the same time, by stressing her conviction that there was a purpose in these events even though it was not clear at that stage, the social worker aimed to convey to Mrs D a sense of hopefulness. Encouragement was communicated through the worker's conviction that Mrs D's difficult situation would not be endured in vain.

10 The worker continued in her work of assessing the situation.

Record   *Comment*

and a tranquilliser and they then
went to sleep. Mrs D said, 'He thinks
tranquillisers help everything' and
laughed. The worker, laughingly,
said how much easier life would be
if pills would put everything right
[11].

11 The worker and patient could
both acknowledge that there were
no easy solutions to the situation.

When asked whether she sometimes
felt frightened, Mrs D said she knew
that she was going to die soon, in
approximately two years, but at the
same time, she felt that 'they' were
going to cure her . . . 'I just want to
live the present circumstances as
they are – to the full' [12]. The
worker nodded and said how understandable that feeling was.

12 The worker noted Mrs D's realistic awareness alongside of her
hope that the situation would
change.

Towards the end of the interview,
the worker summed up that Mrs D
found herself in a difficult situation,
that she felt angry at times, and that
she was drawing fairly firmly upon
her self-discipline in order to cope
[13].

13 The worker drew on the assumption that once the patient understood the situation, she was in a
better position to control or
maintain it.

After the worker had obtained some
identifying details, she worked on
setting a contract. She offered to see
Mrs D from time to time when she
attended the clinic. She also invited
Mrs D to contact her if she ever felt
she needed her services. Mrs D responded with: 'I don't need you.
Anything you say can't make it
better. I'm doing this to help you.
But if you are ever near my home,
do come and have a cup of tea. I'll
talk to you any time' [14].

14 The worker noted that it was important to Mrs D to stress that
she was not dependent; she could

Record   *Comment*

give something to the social worker too. The mutuality of the relationship was important to her. Mrs D's offer of tea might have been a disguised request for the social worker to come and visit her. She could not yet admit that she needed help, but if the social worker offered it in a non-threatening way, that would be acceptable to her.

She said this in a friendly fashion, so the worker thanked her, but did not deal with these feelings [15].

15 The worker considered, on reflection, that she should have dealt with the discomfort Mrs D experienced when in a dependent position. On the other hand, this action might have provoked threat and resistance in Mrs D. The worker's need to build up a caseload, at a time when few referrals were forthcoming, had thus prevailed. The difficulty of rendering a social work service to patients who are not motivated to seek help is apparent.

EVALUATION

The doctor has described Mrs D as 'angry, but with humour'; questioning; an unusual patient who is not easy to pass off when she questions'. He thought she did not know of her secondary malignancies, but had had suspicions from time to time. At that time she had been told (unrealistically) that her chest was clear.

The social worker assessed Mrs D's awareness to be ambivalent; she knew about her forthcoming death but nevertheless held hopes for the future. She seemed to accept the fact of her dying intellectually rather than emotionally. There was little emotion in her tone at all, except when expressing anger. She was, however, partially aware of this factor. She was not permitting herself to feel anything, because a controlled expression of feeling seemed beyond her. She might be overwhelmed if she allowed herself to feel the full impact of her plight.

Mrs D was not without insight; for example, she admitted her stubbornness and impatience to have things done her way. She was also aware of her cleanliness and methodical ways, but it was too early to focus on her rigidity and control. Mrs D was unlikely to request social work intervention in the future but was likely to make use of it if it was made available to her. At that stage she was not in need of intensive social work aid.

Mrs D appeared to be a patient who was trying to cope with the knowledge of her forthcoming death, and was showing (healthy) reactions which confirmed the difficulty of the psychological tasks involved in the terminal crisis: ambivalence, anger, depression and, at that stage, only intellectual acceptance of the situation. Mrs D might move into a stage of more intense anger as she continued in her adjustment to the situation.

The social worker planned to see Mrs D three-weekly at the chemotherapy clinic, to maintain contact with her, to offer her support, to let her set the pace and so control some aspects of the relationships, and to permit her expression of anger and other emotions as she worked on her crisis situation.

Terminal crisis work as described so far draws on several theories, techniques and tasks of social work counselling. In addition to these, I see the social worker's terminal crisis work embodying a number of tasks that are special to the situation in that they correspond to the dying person's adjustment to his circumstances. These tasks include:

1 facilitating the patient's progress through successive emotional stages of adjustment to death;
2 responding to the terminal patient's growing awareness of his condition;
3 aiding the patient to balance hope and fear;
4 facilitating the reversal and relinquishing processes involved in terminal adjustment;
5 ensuring unimpeded detachment from human relationships;
6 providing a climate in which spiritual issues may be explored.

Among those terminal patients who require social work aid, the nature of their terminal difficulty is likely to be fairly specific. Since few patients will struggle with all areas of their terminal adjustment, it is unlikely that any patients will require the social worker to carry out all these terminal crisis work tasks in response.

1 *Facilitating the patient's progress through successive emotional stages of adjustment to death*
One ongoing social work task inherent in terminal crisis work is facilitating the patient's progress through various psychosocial stages of adjustment to death. These six stages have been discussed in Chapter 2. The social worker's response to each of them merits some consideration.

Responding to denial. During the denial stage of adjustment to death, the social worker may either enable the patient to let go his need of denial, that is, to become cognitively and, later, emotionally aware of impending death, or she may choose to support the patient's defence of denial.

Much controversy reigns as to which technique is more helpful in the terminal situation. Heusinkveld (1972) represents one extreme of this continuum in suggesting that the caregiver ought not only to support, but also to reinforce the patient's denial. At the other extreme, Kübler-Ross (1970a) suggests that the patient should be helped to modify or relinquish the defence of denial in favour of a more realistic method of adjusting to the situation. Like Kübler-Ross, I deplore the practice of reinforcing denial, as it often amounts to offering false reassurance, and does not aid the patient in reaching an acceptance of his situation. On the contrary, it entrenches him in the unproductive, fear-filled, non-coping and lonely position of not adjusting to dying.

Saunders (1976) reminds us that the question to ask in response to denial is *not* 'should the doctor tell?' or 'does the patient have the right to know?' but 'how can I enable the patient to tell me, if and when he is ready to do so?' Another response to denial, suggested by a psychiatrist colleague, is to say something like: 'My task is to discuss dying with you . . . I may be wrong; if so, nothing will be lost. If I am right, you will be prepared . . .' Or, put another way:

Caregiver: I think you need a lawyer.
Patient: Not yet . . . I am not dying.
Caregiver: I may be wrong, but I still think you need a lawyer . . .

This form of approach has several merits. It avoids deceit and false reassurances; it does not take away hope, and it reinforces the caregiver's fallibility. On the other hand, it may prove a little too blunt for some patients who are denying the situation. The social worker's response to relatives who, albeit unwittingly, frequently adopt denying techniques in the terminal situation is to present a contrast and maintain an open communication system both with the patient and the family.

The social worker's suggested response to denial may thus be summed up as follows. She needs to respect that patient's need for denial and to move at his pace. She can then let the patient lead the way and guide her as to his readiness to drop this defence. She need not reinforce or introduce denial into the terminal situation but can remain neutral, willing and able to acknowledge the reality of impending death as and when the patient indicates *his* readiness to move on to one of the next stages of adjustment. And, finally, she needs so to word her responses as to leave room for some hope, but not necessarily for hope of a cure.

Case illustration 12: a patient's use of denial and the social worker's response

THE INITIAL CONTACT (in the flat of the patient's son)

Mr A, a 64-year-old widower, developed bronchial carcinoma after a fairly healthy life. When talking to the social worker of his earlier life, it became evident that Mr A had used denial as a defence against many life crises. For example, when his wife died twenty years previously, he had 'not let it upset' him or his routine. He told the worker, 'I looked after our son who was only 2 years old at the time, and that and my work kept me too busy to think about my wife's death'. From these words it appeared that Mr A had not permitted himself to mourn the loss and had hardly acknowledged that he had any cause to grieve at all. Since then he had lived an asocial, hermit-like existence, denying his need for other people, while protesting that he was occupied and happy enough.

Since Mr A was unready to engage in any new meaningful relationships as a result of incomplete grief work, he aimed at self-sufficiency – which he conceived of as control of his feelings and a determination not to give way. This defence pattern was expressed chiefly in the form of denying that any life events troubled him. He said of many issues: 'It does not bother me.'

Once Mr A became terminally ill he responded, characteristically, with denial. He explained that he 'had had a gland removed from the lung', and that he expected to recover once the treatment (radiotherapy) had been completed. He said his present situation did 'not bother him'. For example, on account of his illness Mr A was no longer able to go to work, had given up the independence of his own home, had moved into the flat of his newly-wedded son, was left unattended in this flat all day and was isolated by his son and daughter-in-law at weekends, and responded to all these events as 'just one of those things'.

Mr A hardly complained or discussed his illness at all. In response to the social worker's persevering questioning, he answered monosyllabically that he was in pain, was not eating and felt nauseous. He disclosed nothing more of what he was feeling or suffering, saying that it did not help to 'perform' or to 'complain'. These remarks suggested that Mr A's earlier efforts to express his feelings had not had the results he desired. Consequently, the defence of 'not complaining' (that is a defence of control and denial of feeling) had been reinforced.

At the first interview with the social worker Mr A had denied many issues. At that stage it was difficult to assess whether he was using the defence of denial, because (a) he could not yet tolerate the reality of his difficult situation (see Kübler-Ross, 1970a); (b) he was testing out the social worker's reactions to his terminal situation, before exposing his difficulties (see Weisman, 1972a); or (c) significant others in his environment had been unable to tolerate thoughts of dying and death; consequently Mr A now expected the worker to respond in the same way. He probably thought that in order to maintain the social worker's interest and care, he would respond as he thought she expected him to do, that is, with control and denial (Weisman's theory). In the latter two situations the denial would have been (consciously) controlled by Mr A; if the first condition applied denial would have occurred as an unconscious, involuntary defence mechanism. Either way, it was clear at that stage that this patient needed to deny and that he did not wish for fuller awareness.

THE SECOND INTERVIEW (two weeks later)

During the second consultation session with the social worker Mr A was able to acknowledge that he felt that he was intruding on his son and daughter-in-law by living with them so soon after they were married. This admission indicated slight progress, in that Mr A no longer needed to deny *all* his feelings.

THE THIRD INTERVIEW (four weeks later)

By the third interview, when Mr A was suddenly seriously ill and confined to bed, he consistently denied all feeling again. Between each counselling session, the worker had tried to initiate further, more frequent contact with Mr A. She visited or phoned weekly, but was told that the patient was out, had gone back to work, or, when he was gravely ill, she was told that he did not wish to see any visitors. Therefore some weeks elapsed before she was able to see him again.

THE FOURTH INTERVIEW (two weeks later)

The fourth interview took place once Mr A was somewhat recovered, and he was dressed and sitting in the lounge. During this session he agreed with the social worker's remarks that he might be wondering what his illness was about, and that in such a situation one might sometimes wonder whether one would get better at all. He then looked down, sat quietly, said no more, and the subject was changed.

The last reaction was thought to constitute slight progress: even though Mr A could not yet admit to verbalise his thoughts about dying, at least he no longer denied them. The improved response was made possible, in Weisman's sense, by the worker's demonstrated ability to tolerate thoughts of dying and death. At the same time it would seem, in terms of Kübler-Ross's theory, that Mr A was himself beginning to find it possible to tolerate the thought of his impending death. Somehow, the event was no longer totally unacceptable. The topic nevertheless remained a painful one for Mr A. Consequently once he showed no willingness to communicate further on that topic, the social worker respected his defence and the need to move at his own pace and she therefore changed the subject for him.

THE FIFTH INTERVIEW (two and a half weeks later)

During the final interview, when Mr A was at the point of death, he again demonstrated his wish to remain in control of the situation by ensuring that the worker did not intend to remain with him for long before permitting her to sit down at all.

He told the worker that he knew he was dying by saying simply, 'It's really serious now . . .' The worker responded by acknowledging that his situation was serious. Since he was too ill to talk more, a short silence followed during which Mr A looked anxious. Remembering that he wished to remain in control of his feelings, the worker again changed the subject for him. He died five days later.

Responding to isolation. Terminal caregivers usually aim to combat, or minimize, the dying person's sense of isolation (Saunders, 1966b). In responding to the dying patient's isolation, the worker's mere presence in the terminal situation or, in the terms of Salzberger-Wittenberg (1970), her ability to 'hold' the emotions which the patient experiences – in contrast to others who have withdrawn from this difficult situation – carries a conviction that the patient's terminal situation is bearable. In 'holding' the patient's emotions in this way, encouragement and support are communicated to him. This dynamic of containing the patient's feelings is demonstrated with Mr B (pp. 70–1) and Mr N (pp. 51–6).

The social worker's response to the terminal patient's isolation thus consists of acknowledging his insular position. She can enable him to verbalise his feelings of aloneness, resentment and envy and his fear of future rejection. Whenever realistically possible, he can be assured that he will receive adequate care, that he will not be permitted to suffer unduly and that he will not be abandoned. At the same time, the social worker works with the patient's caregivers to make them aware of the part they play in intensifying or diminishing his sense of isolation.

To the patient who isolates himself in order to protect his relatives from his awareness of dying, one social work response can be to enable him to verbalise these feelings to her, while supporting his efforts to present a brave front to his family. A word of caution is, however, indicated here. In responding to the terminal patient's sense of isolation, the social worker needs to be wary of overidentifying with the patient at the expense of his family. To ally herself too closely with the patient may alienate the family. It may also antagonise a family which is jealously guarding its relationship with the loved one who is soon to depart. The social worker, therefore, needs to remain available to and in close contact with both the patient and his family throughout the terminal period.

Case illustration 13: an isolated patient and the social worker's response

Mr B, a young man of 26 years with disseminated carcinoma of the spine and nerves of the lower half of his body, lay paralysed in hospital after being ill for two years. He was unmarried, the elder son of a widower. He had always been withdrawn and not very communicative.

For six weeks, Mr B had hovered on the brink of death: he had lost all movement and control over his lower abdomen, legs, feet and back. The growth on his spine prevented his lying on his back. Bedsores, which daily increased in size, restricted his positioning still further. He was turned two-hourly, as he could no longer move himself. The open bedsores gave off an unpleasant odour. Pain was constant. Medical and nursing staff found it difficult to talk to him and gradually withdrew all but essential, meaningless, contact with him.

Mr B's only visitor had been his father, who came dutifully every evening. At this time, Mr B's father isolated him further by visiting only every second night, saying that it was 'too much' for him to come daily. By way of justification, Mr B's father said that he did not 'feel very well at present'. The social worker assessed this decreased contact to be a communication that the patient's father could no longer bear the situation. He was therefore avoiding the situation, as an act of self-defence. Although this motive appeared to have crossed Mr B's mind, he denied feeling rejected or sad about his father's less frequent visits.

Over the next few weeks Mr B began to isolate himself still further, in order to test his caregiver's sincerity and dependability. He feigned fatigue or sleep either as the social worker approached or after some minutes of her visit. Thus she often had to return to Mr B's ward more than once a day in order to see him when he was 'less tired'. On some days he said that he did not feel like talking at all, thus rebuffing her approach. When she offered just to sit at his bedside for a while, while he dozed, he refused this offer. When he did agree to a short visit he was unresponsive and denied all former insights, so that the worker was made to feel impotent and inadequate. In similar manner, he became an 'unrewarding case' to many members of staff, many of whom withdrew their contact, leaving Mr B yet more alone.

At the same time, Mr B appeared to manipulate one team member against another by saying to the chaplain that the social worker talked too much, to the social worker that the chaplain never had time to talk when he visited and to the nursing auxiliary that he did not appreciate the visits of either the social worker or the chaplain. These tactics had the effect of testing his care-givers' commitment to the full. It was extremely difficult to continue a contact with a patient who seemed so unresponsive and immobilised. Many staff members asked themselves whether it was worth continuing with 'an obviously hopeless case' and decided instead, partly in response to their own feelings of discomfort, to offer their services in more rewarding avenues.

It was only the (difficult) recognition that Mr B's desperation drove him to use such self-defeating tactics that enabled the social worker to continue to visit him through this period of partially self-inflicted isolation. The worker understood that these actions were a sign of Mr B's loss of self esteem and his inability to bear the situation. His behaviour was unconsciously adopted to elicit some reassurance of his worth and acceptability. Consequently the worker was not rebuffed. She could have tried to help Mr B to verbalise his isolation and to understand that his contradictory communications to different caregivers were a plea for continued care from them all. With this very withdrawn patient, however, the worker estimated that what was said was less important than her continued presence. She therefore continued to visit Mr B, although relatively little verbal counselling was attempted. Instead, the worker's presence offered a 'holding' element to the situation. Her ability to bear it aided Mr B to some extent in containing his desperation.

Mr B remained isolated and withdrawn until his death a month later.

Responding to anger. As will be shown in the case of Mrs C (below) the social worker's task with the angry patient is to understand that the anger is not intended personally but that it expresses envy of and resentment towards those who represent the health and functioning which the patient is in the process of losing. Consequently, if the worker enables the patient to ventilate his anger, encourages his questioning and demands, facilitates his exploration of the possible meaning of the situation and tolerates the hostility, he will gradually need to act out less of his anger, will be able to understand and contain it himself and become less demanding and critical and easier to manage. Answers like 'Why *not* you?' '*Is* there something in your life that you feel merits punishment?' or 'What is it that would help you now?' are likely to prove useful in introducing such discussion.

Where relatives are angry in their efforts to understand what is happening the social worker can aid them to understand the patient's behaviour and not react to it. At the same time she can enable them to ventilate and explore their own angry feelings. Where anger is vented against God the worker may enable the patient (or family member) to explore his feelings concerning religion and how God could helpfully be drawn into the situation.

Case illustration 14: an angry patient and the social worker's response

Mrs C, a 42-year-old lady with carcinoma of the ovary, was admitted to hospital at a time when the possibility of a spread of the condition appeared evident to the doctors. She was admitted for full investigation and assessment with regard to future treatment.

She had been told two years previously when the disease was first discovered that she had cancer. She had thought, however, that after surgical removal of one ovary she had been cured. She had nevertheless received chemotherapy ever since that operation. Now, two years later, thoughts of cancer (and of death) presented themselves again. Mrs C's suspicions were confirmed when another doctor discussed her condition with her. She responded with fury, as she had come to believe during the intervening years that she had been cured. For valid reasons no tests or X-rays had been carried out during the intervening period. Now she focused on the lack of routine examination, calling it 'neglect and inefficiency'. After two years of painful, unpleasant treatment she felt that nothing had been achieved and that 'they [the treatment team] were back to square one'. Mrs C railed against her doctor saying that he was silly not to have warned her sooner. He had done himself a wrong in not telling her that the carcinoma had not been completely arrested, even though his motive might have been not to hurt her. She felt that now they were so angry with each other they were unable to communicate, and he was as hurt by her anger as she was on account of his avoidance of her.

The relationship between Mrs C and her doctor worsened. She was angry, critical and complaining and he avoided her in this frame of mind. She became yet more angry at being 'snubbed' by him. She also felt let down, disappointed and puzzled by his behaviour. Mrs C focused her anger solely on her doctor, thereby localising it and avoiding the pain of exploring this emotion in relation to her dying. Later she became critical of other patients in the ward and complained about their behaviour, the hospital's treatment, her care and the food until many of the staff, and some patients, were antagonised. It was only once Mrs C had moved into the bargaining and depression stages of her illness that she permitted the social worker to reach the fears and feelings which had prompted the long spell of anger.

In response, the social worker helped Mrs C to verbalise her anger and to ventilate these intense feelings as often as she needed to, without fear of retaliation and without fear that the worker would take it all personally. The worker's ability to hold the aggression helped Mrs C to manage some of her emotion for herself and freed her of her fears of her anger and its destructiveness. Only then could Mrs C begin to explore the cause of her pent-up anger. In this way Mrs C was mobilised again and was enabled to progress in her death work.

She moved through a period of depression during the following two months, and died a week after she had reached a calm acceptance of her situation.

Mrs C's anger mirrors Kübler-Ross's description in many aspects: it was manifest as hostility, rebuffing the person whose aid was most needed at that time, that is, the doctor. In saying that the doctor was hurt by their breakdown in communication Mrs C seemed to imply retaliation, that is, she almost wanted him also to be hurt. Her anger was expressed in the form of complaints and criticism and was used as a plea in which she was asking the staff to notice her plight, to understand and to help her. For a long time she rebuffed attempts to help her examine the underlying cause of her anger, and kept potential helpers at bay.

Responding to bargaining. The social worker's role during the bargaining stage of the terminal crisis is to listen to the bargaining to understand and respond to its importance and to learn from such discussions what the patient most hopes and fears in his present situation. Wherever possible, the bargains should be permitted, as their effects will enable the patient to move on towards acceptance. Another useful response is to ask whom the patient would like to put in his place. This may give a clue as to who the hated or envied one is – in fantasy or reality. The social worker's availability to both the patient and his relatives is important during this stage of dying work as the family may be as busily engaged in its bargaining in the situation as the patient is. If the patient bargains with God the social worker may need to provide opportunities to discuss some spiritual aspects of the situation, as the bargainer will be involved in some way in a conscious relationship with God.

Case illustration 15: a terminal patient bargains for more time

Mrs D, a 43-year-old wife and mother with disseminated carcinoma, wished to be at home with her family for Christmas. Although in need of hospitalised care early in December, she resisted readmission to hospital, saying that if she went into hospital she would never come out again. She bargained that if she could only be with her family till Christmas time, she would then be content to die.

Understanding the patient's wish to fulfil this last duty as a wife and mother, the social worker responded by supporting Mrs D's attempts to remain at home, despite grave deterioration in her physical condition. She assisted Mrs D with some necessary practical arrangements and negotiated to have Mrs D readmitted to hospital at short notice, if necessary. She also explained the importance of Mrs D's wish to remain at home to her family and aided them in ventilating their concern over her condition and their fears of inadequacy in nursing her satisfactorily at home.

Mrs D remained at home, spent a quiet Christmas with her family, and died the following day. The bargain had been executed on both sides.

This striking example of bargaining occurred very shortly before death. In most of her cases, Kübler-Ross (1970a), has observed bargaining earlier on in the terminal crisis and especially preceding a period of depression. Mrs D, however, experienced these two emotions in reverse order (see case illustration 16, p. 74).

Responding to depression. The effective way to respond to terminal depression is to permit it. Skill is needed here simply in order not to block its expression. Both the patient and his relatives require that the social worker understands the naturalness of their depression concerning what is to be lost. She can then help them to acknowledge their sadness. Much of this work may take place non-verbally. The social worker's ability simply to be there, to contain these often intense emotions and to tolerate the patient's anguished feelings constitutes her catalytic function of enabling the patient and his family to move towards acceptance. She may need to stay there until the patient withdraws, as he will, when he is ready to meet what is to come.

Working with dying people who are depressed also frequently leads to discussion of the religious or spiritual issues involved in the situation (Hinton, 1968a; Kübler-Ross, 1974; Saunders, 1976). The patient may initiate such discussion or, in some cases, the worker may sensitively offer such topics for consideration (Leslie, 1960). The patient's response will determine whether or not to pursue the subject further.

Case illustration 16: a period of terminal depression and the social worker's response

Mrs D, a 43-year-old wife and mother, had carcinoma of the breast and secondary malignancy in her lungs. After three years of illness a further malignancy was discovered in her liver, indicating disseminated carcinoma. She was admitted to hospital for assessment of her condition and to plan her future treatment. Prior to this episode, Mrs D had remained fairly well for two years. She realised at the time of admission to hospital that this further area of contamination would prove fatal and that it was merely a question of time before she died. Her depression was observable from the time that she was informed that she would be admitted to hospital. She was sad as she wondered whether she would ever be healed and whether her husband and son would experience difficulties without her.

Once in hospital Mrs D said that she was not yet sick enough to die nor well enough to live; that she felt lost, like a green pea in a whole sea, and that she would sell her soul in order to have her health back. In these ways she was able to express her sadness, which at that time was tinged with isolation, resentment and bargaining.

In the following weeks, as she worked on her situation, Mrs D often said that she was 'trying to sort herself out'. She wanted to get better and to do all the things she used to do. She communicated her awareness of impending death to her husband and discussed the situation with him. Soon after she told the social worker that it had 'to happen to all couples sooner or later; so it's happening to us sooner.' At that time she distracted her depressed feelings and reacted to her loss of control over her situation by planning how her family might live after her death.*

Depression was evident in Mrs D's flat tone, especially while talking of emotional issues. She complained of feeling listless and useless and of having no energy. She felt she would be an nuisance at home and consequently chose to remain in hospital, even over weekends. Pain increased her general debility and depression.

Mrs D's appreciation of impending loss was evident in remarks concerning her inability to go shopping, to do the weekly washing, or even to manage

* See case illustration 23: terminal crisis work with a relative of a patient, pp. 97–103.

her own toilette while in hospital. These activities constituted the control of her home and family, that is, the usual, routine things with which she had filled her days while well. Now she seemed to be mourning the loss of that control and of her former self-esteem which had accompanied it. She regretted sleeping so much, saying that she did not want to sleep her life away, but that it was terrible not to have energy.

Hopeless depression was obvious when, one day, Mrs D said that she felt she had one foot in the grave and one on a banana peel, and that she had lived like this for so long that she felt that if she crawled out of one, she would only slip on the other. The hospital staff also observed and commented on Mrs D's depression at this stage.

This example shows depression as an intense, pervasive experience, appropriate to the process of adjusting to loss and separation. Mrs D's realistic approach to her situation enabled her, with the help of her family and the social worker, to move through depression, once more back to bargaining and then on to the final stage of adjustment: acceptance.

Responding to acceptance. Basically the response that acceptance draws forth is our acknowledgement of it. At this stage the patient hardly needs any further psychosocial help although he will of course require considerable physical care. More practically, however, the social worker needs to slow down in order to respond effectively to this final stage of dying. Presenting an unhurried and unfrightened approach, she could continue to visit the patient daily until he dies. Communication is likely to be non-verbal and to consist of a silent sharing of the situation. Physical contact, for example, holding the patient's hand, is often reassuring to him. He needs to be assured of the social worker's presence and availability in case he should wish to speak. Her role changes from active participant to silent companion to the patient, while her role as counsellor to the family remains active. She now needs to focus on the family members, who often find the final stages of a terminal situation difficult to endure and merit help both in their own right and in order to prevent interference with the patient's dying (Kübler-Ross, 1970a). The social worker's response to acceptance may also take the form, as in other stages of adjustment to death, of providing an avenue for the consideration of spiritual issues, which will be discussed further on in this chapter.

Thus to summarise, the task of facilitating progress towards acceptance requires that the social worker understands the dynamics and sequence of the feeling inherent in the terminal situation; she needs to identify the stages of adjustment in which the patient is currently engaged; to decode his behaviour to the patient himself, his relatives and his caregivers; to handle the emotions as they would be handled in any other life crisis; to remain in the situation in order to act as catalyst to the patient's conscious and sometimes verbal progression towards acceptance; and she needs to work with the family, as well as the patient, in order to help them all to master this life crisis. (Kübler-Ross, 1970b). Additional examples of this terminal crisis work task appear throughout the text.

By contrast we should note that some patients do not make progress in their terminal crisis work, despite social work intervention. For example:

Case illustration 17: a patient who made no progress in her terminal crisis work, despite social work intervention

Mrs O, 55 years of age, a wife and mother of two late adolescent sons, was a professional person, who had worked during most of her married life and had gained much gratification from the esteem and status that came to her in her professional capacity. Mrs O had had a slight physical disability, to which her major response had been denial. She was described to the worker as 'a denier in everything'. When she became terminally ill her denial prevailed.

Mrs O's family had been angry about her impending death, but had had difficulty in expressing anger as they had also used denial as a protective defence. Hence they said that there was no need of social work aid.

Issues of control became increasingly important to Mrs O, as she struggled not to 'give in', and to maintain her denial. Since she denied that she was in need at all, she did not allow the social work consultations to become meaningful to her. For example, she tried to turn the worker's home visits into social events.

Although Mrs O needed to deny her terminal situation she was troubled by her family's refusal to acknowledge her plight. At one point therefore in her desperation to break through her own and her family's contrived nonchalance she underwent a minor psychotic episode, for which she was admitted to the psychiatric ward of the hospital. During that period communications in the family became yet more confused, hostile, guilty and deceptive. Again the social worker's intervention was rebuffed and she was treated as a social visitor. Nevertheless she maintained her contact with Mrs O and her family, trying, with little success, to intersperse something meaningful into her relationship with them.

Mrs O died in agony of body and mind. She was described by a hospital doctor as having died in a dehumanised state.

Although she did not see Mrs O frequently, the social worker did not withdraw her service altogether. Thus difficulties in Mrs O's life, during which she had denied many issues and defied professional intervention, culminated in grave difficulties in dying.

2 *Responding to the terminal patient's growing awareness of his condition*

Terminal crisis work invariably involves some response to the dying person's growing awareness of impending death. In our discussion on reacting to denial we have already dealt with the handling of the patient who is not yet acknowledging his awareness. In order to respond, the caregiver needs to assess whether the person really wants to know that he is dying. There is no easy method of ascertaining whether the patient who asks for information does in fact want it. But I firmly believe that if we listen the patient will give us enough consistent clues to indicate his readiness, or otherwise, to assimilate the information he is requesting. Listening to facts, feelings, patterns, repetitions and timing, and noting the patient's choice of listener remain our major tools for this assessment (Saunders, 1966b). The related issue of 'telling the patient' has aroused much controversy in the field of terminal care. Thus let me repeat that it is the contention of many writers, and myself, that the task of the caregiver is not one of telling the patient that he is dying, but rather of communicating with him in such a manner that he may feel free, if and when *he* is ready, to tell her of his growing awareness of impending death (Hinton, 1968a; Kübler-Ross, 1970a; Saunders, 1976). Each case needs to be assessed on its own merits.

Responding to awareness therefore involves communication and particularly listening. In this way the patient is enabled to verbalise his fears and to talk of dying in hypothetical terms, as a prelude to confronting death work in reality. Using this technique the worker is able to facilitate the patient's preparation for death without having to confirm or deny that he is in fact dying. Nor do the patient's defences need to be broken down; if the threat is first confronted at a distance the patient will drop his protective defences when he is ready. This technique also enables the patient to maintain his hopefulness which, as Kübler-Ross (1972) stresses, is vital in sound terminal care.

Since Cramond (1970) has found that 80 per cent of terminal patients know that they are dying and wish to talk of it, while 80 per cent of doctors do not permit their patients to talk of it, the social worker's response is simply not to block the communication. In other words, she should ensure that the patient too does not believe that she, like so many other caregivers, expects him to deny his plight and feign non-complaining cheerfulness (Pilsecker, 1975). Again this position may be difficult for the social worker to adopt if the rest of the team members use denying techniques. The views of the doctor and nurse are thus significant in determining how best to respond to the patient on this – and other – issues. Since awareness of death fluctuates throughout the terminal period, communication on this topic is likely to require frequent repetition until the patient acknowledges consciously that he is dying.

Case illustration 18: terminal crisis work focusing on communication concerning the patient's awareness of impending death

Mr L, a 57-year-old widower, had carcinoma of the bronchus. He had had severe arthritis for thirty-five years, so that it seemed to him that he had been ill for nearly all his life. A year after the discovery of his malignant condition, he was readmitted to hospital for investigation. It appeared that the malignancy had spread to his stomach. He suffered abdominal pain and discomfort, vomited frequently and could keep little food down. The ward sister did not know of his malignant condition, and he was not receiving any medication for pain. Concerning Mr L's awareness of his condition, his married daughter had told the worker that he had never been told that he had cancer. He had once asked, but upon instruction from a hospital doctor his family had answered in the negative. He had not asked again. His daughter said that he had found out by seeing the medical term written on an unemployment document which was completed for him by a doctor in the hospital. Mr L had looked up the words in a dictionary, had come to tell his daughter, but had never mentioned it again. Mr L's daughter thought that he had not been shocked or upset at discovering that he had cancer, as he had probably suspected it all along.

EXTRACT FROM FOURTH INTERVIEW WITH MR L (in hospital)

Aim: to establish more intensive contact with Mr L as his condition worsened and to aid him in his terminal work

Record	*Comment*
Mr L smiled welcome to the worker. He looked much thinner and weaker than when last the worker had seen him. He said he felt better since being in hospital. He thought that his condition was improving, because he had managed to eat a little. He acknowledgd that he had made 'slow progress' (towards recovery) since his operation a year previously, but, he reassured himself, 'it takes time'.	
The worker noted Mr L's apparent non-awareness of his situation [1].	1 It was difficult at that stage to estimate which theory applied to Mr L's use of denial. In denying his deteriorating condition he was also denying his impending death. In terms of Weisman's (1972a) theory, in order to maintain his

Record

Comment

relationship with the worker he would control any mention of non-recovery until he was more sure of her readiness to discuss dying. Or, in terms of Kübler-Ross's (1974) theory, Mr L was emotionally unable at that time to acknowledge that his deterioration implied that he was never going to recover, as the thought was too threatening to him.

The worker helped Mr L to focus on his feelings concerning his illness. He said that at times progress was so slow that he began to give up hope. He dealt with these depressed feelings by sleeping and hoped that he would feel better on waking, which he often did. He acknowledged that fairly often he felt 'down in the dumps', but that he fought against this feeling for his own sake and for the sake of his family, who were unable to tolerate his depression. Mr L's son-in-law seemed especially upset when Mr L was depressed. The family responded by trying to jolly Mr L along. He was aware of his family's distress, as a result of which he tried not to talk about his illness at all [2]. Consequently he bore his situation alone, and acknowledged that that was not always easy to manage.

2 Mr L's established pattern of functioning became apparent: he was obedient, in exchange for which he could expect care. For example, he noted that his family was upset by any reference to his condition and so, obediently, he tried not to talk about it; in return he was cared for by them.

The worker verbalised some of these difficulties for Mr L and clarified that great effort was required in order to bear the situation alone [3].

3 The worker took an active role with this passive terminal patient. In recognising Mr L's efforts to be brave, the worker was meeting his need for reward: since his

Record

Comment

life-long obedience had apparently not been rewarded, it was appropriate that she should reward his efforts.

The worker related the difficulties of Mr L's terminal situation to difficulties in his earlier life [4]. He acknowledged that he had had a hard life and told the worker that his father had died when he was only 14. He had had to go out to work at that age and had worked ever since.

4 This step enabled Mr L to talk of his problems, to connect similarities and to perceive patterns in his behaviour and situation.

The worker asked what had caused his father's death [5]. Mr L answered that he had had cancer of the throat. The worker asked whether anyone else in his family had had cancer. Then Mr L said: 'I think I have too . . .', to which the worker replied, 'I'm sure you must think that at times . . .' [6] '. . . what makes you think so?' [7].

5 By presenting obvious connections to Mr L the worker aimed to communicate her willingness to confront terminal issues, to help him to confront his reality and to discuss dying, if he should so wish.

6 The worker acknowledged the sanity of Mr L's deduction without blocking his freedom to speak further upon the subject. At the same time, however, she did not confirm or deny the suspicion.

7 With this question the worker put Mr L in touch with the reality of his deduction and invited him to ventilate his fears.

Mr L: This is not getting better. This feeling so weak, and the pain . . . I saw a doctor's letter once, and read it, and looked up the word, and asked my family, but they said 'No' . . .
W: But you still think so?
Mr L: Yes . . .
W: If it *were* so, what would you feel [8]?

8 The worker again did not confirm the diagnosis but enabled Mr L further ventilation of his thoughts and feelings concerning his condition.

Record

Mr L: It's all right... [9] I'm pleased to die... I've had my life. The children are grown up and can look after themselves now... Once *they* were OK, my body gave up... [10)

W: You've worked hard to bring them up, haven't you [11]?

Mr L: Yes.
W: Do you have any regrets [12]?

Mr L: Yes, I regret my hard life ... I *tried* to better myself... [13].

W: But it was hard... [14].
Mr L: Yes.

The worker asked if Mr L was tired, but he said not, and invited her to go on.

Comment

9 It was always a surprise to the worker to hear how easily and gladly some patients anticipated death. On such occasions she wondered why caregivers found it so difficult to discuss dying with their patients.

10 The worker was not sure how to relate this insightful remark to the rest of Mr L's functioning.

11 The worker again offered a reward for Mr L's efforts. She recognised his efforts and, since hard work is considered a positive social value, she was recognising his social worth.

12 The worker gave Mr L another opportunity to express any negative feelings which he might have been experiencing.

13 Mr L took the opportunity; he sounded indignant and angry at life's hardship.

14 The worker offered understanding and support of his anger.

The rest of the interview centred on Mr L's feelings concerning his situation and his spiritual ideas at that time.

When the worker said goodbye Mr L said more than once how nice it was of her to come to see him and that he had not expected to see her. He twice thanked her for her visit.

EVALUATION

The worker left Mr L feeling that the interview had been a useful one. Her relationship with Mr L had been deepened. He had willingly and consciously been able to make use of the worker's presence to work on his situation. At first Mr L had needed to deny his terminal condition, but he was able to drop this defence as the consultation session wore on and he was assured that the worker could tolerate the truth with him.

The worker assessed that Mr L was fairly near to death, willing to work on his terminal situation and amenable to social work, and she thus planned to see him intensively from then on.

This illustration highlights the social worker's response to the patient's awareness of his condition and shows how the patient's terminal crisis work may be facilitated by effective, open communication between himself and the caregiver.

3   Aiding the patient to balance hope and fear

A third task for the social worker is aiding the patient to balance his hope and fear in the terminal crisis. The patient will need social work help in order to explore both these feelings courageously and make some sense of them. Since what may be thought of as a fear of death is in fact often a fear concerning some related aspect of life, this task is likely to involve uncovering the connections, counselling in those areas (Rosenthal, 1963) and helping the patient to maintain hope by finding some meaning in his suffering while at the same time ensuring that he does not merely hope unrealistically for a cure. Equally she can ensure that he is permitted as full an expression and exploration of his fears as he needs. She can also help the patient to modify and adapt his hopes and fears to each stage of adjustment. Examples of handling hope and fears appear throughout the text. See especially illustrations of Mr L, whose fears diminished as hopelessness was dispelled and his perception of the meaning of his suffering increased.

4   Facilitating the reversal and relinquishing processes involved in terminal adjustment

A fourth area of social work response consists in enabling the patient to reverse former physical survival processes and so to engage in the work of moving from dying to death itself.

Since the patient's task of relinquishing various aspects of life is closely intertwined with the reversal process which precedes it the social worker may respond to both areas of dying work simultaneously. Consequently we discuss them together here. It is difficult to prescribe how the social worker should perform these two closely associated tasks. Current literature offers no specific guidelines. Hence I suggest that the caregiver's understanding of the dynamics of the terminal crisis may have to suffice as her guide. Her task, then, is to identify the patient's area of conflict, assist him to acknowledge the difficulty and then counsel in that area, as she might in any other stage of life.

Unresolved conflicts in life may prevent peace in dying (Rosenthal, 1957 and 1963). Accordingly, one way of facilitating the patient's reversal and relinquishing processes is to focus on the relevant problem areas of his life. The cause of his difficulty in resolving his terminal crisis is likely to be found among issues of control, dependency or autonomy and in the regrets, disappointments or guilt which dying has provoked. As in other social work counselling the social worker can help the patient to review his past, to try to perceive and understand some of its patterns and, in this way, to relate his life to what he is presently experiencing in dying.

Case illustration 19: the social worker attempts to facilitate the reversal and relinquishing processes involved in terminal adjustment

Mr H, 51 years old, with carcinoma of the lung, had throughout life fought for independent control of himself and his situation, and had entrenched himself stubbornly into a number of positions in life. For example, for some years he drank heavily. Then through his own self-control he stopped and never drank again.

When dying, Mr H's struggle for control was centred around the problem of breathing. He held fast, forcing himself to breathe either with increasing supplies of oxygen or, later, with conscious control of each breath. In struggling thus, he evaded a reversal of physical survival processes for five months.

While he was engaged in this physical struggle for survival, little energy was released for emotional or spiritual growth. Consequently Mr H showed little movement in these areas during a terminal period of fifteen months.

During a social work interview a month before he died Mr H struggled for breath. He had chest pain and was in distress, as was evidenced by his constant frown and clenched fists. His dishevelled demeanour communicated tension and a determination to fight on.

The worker observed that Mr H was battling and used the term 'giving over' to describe the relinquishing process that was presently required of him. Mr H immediately responded by saying that to his Scottish background 'giving over' was the same as 'giving up', which he was not prepared to do. The worker described the process of giving over as a heroic, courageous act and said that it required great strength to depend on something beyond oneself. She commented that Mr H seemed to see letting go as a cowardly act. He replied that he could understand what she was saying: everyone had to depend on something bigger than himself, but it was not easy for him as he was not used to dependence. The worker acknowledged this difficulty. Then, wanting to encourage Mr H in the relinquishing process, she observed that it appeared to be as difficult for him to hold on as it was to give over his control.

Although Mr H had begun the interview with denial, saying: 'It's flu', he moved towards awareness of the situation and was able to acknowledge that he felt the end was near. He said it was not a pleasant feeling; it was in fact overwhelming to feel that one's own end was in sight. The worker verbalised that it was perhaps Mr H's fear of being overwhelmed (that is, out of control) that made him shrink from death.

Throughout the interview, since Mr H was struggling for breath, the worker helped him to verbalise his feelings by putting them into words for him. He could acknowledge that he was depressed, that he felt sadness and loss and that he had little interest in anything any more. The worker nodded that she understood, and, in an effort to help him to ventilate further, asked if he could say a little more of what he was feeling. At this point, however, his awareness of his impending death became too painful and he withdrew from it by saying that he was not really alert enough to say more. He said he felt like sleeping, and he closed his eyes. The worker responded to this cue and said she would leave him. As a reassurance of her continued availability and care, she said she would see him again a day later.

Mr H's refusal to give over the fight for survival appeared to be linked to his (lack of) spiritual preparation for death. He had come from a somewhat restrictive Christian home. He had broken away from all religious belief, because he had seen so much hypocritical practice, and had lived without faith for most of his life. Now, in dying, he said he still did not believe in God, that life did not continue beyond death and, therefore, he had nothing to fear. Nevertheless, although he refuted religion his wife was a Christian and was concerned for his soul. Consequently the issue of religion was raised from time to time. On most occasions Mr H remained adamant that there was nothing to fear. On one occasion, however, he mused to the social worker that if life did, in fact, continue after death, 'then I'm in for a bad time, aren't I?'

The worker used this remark to focus on Mr H's fear of death, which until then he had consistently denied. She acknowledged that he might be in for a bad time, and reminded him that it was within his power to alter his fate, if he so wished. Mr H. said it was too late to do that, to which the worker responded that it was never too late to change.

Bearing in mind the connection of these two terminal tasks: relinquishing life and spiritual preparation for death, the worker tried to facilitate Mr H's work in both areas simultaneously. It seemed that Mr H would give over only once he was sure that death would not lead to hell. But while he denied God and an after life, he saw no reason to change in order to avoid hell. Then at times when the spiritual dimension of the situation appeared real to him, Mr H shrank from it, saying 'it's too late now'. At other times he denied his fear of death, saying that he feared suffocation, not death itself, Mr H had again entrenched himself in an impasse.

During the worker's twelve subsequent visits to Mr H the themes of giving over, fear of death and the brief span of time still available to him recurred frequently. Each time the same impasse was reached. Each time the worker reaffirmed that although it was difficult to change, it was never too late to do so. But Mr H stubbornly refused to move from his unhappy position. His satisfaction in so doing lay in the realisation that *he* had controlled this situation. However uncomfortable his control might be, at least it had been maintained. He struggled along in this position for four weeks before he died. These conflicts remained unresolved.

This illustration demonstrates the complicated nature of terminal conflicts: while one problem-solving area of dying remains unresolved, the accomplishment of other tasks may be hampered. In Mr H's case, an absence of spiritual preparation for death caused him to fear what might lie beyond death and so to fight on for life. This illustration bears out the statement that patterns of living influence dying (Rosenthal, 1957 and 1963).

Mr H's case also highlights the social worker's response to a terminal conflict. Encouraging the patient to give over has proved to be an ineffective technique. The reason underlying the patient's resistance, feelings and behaviour cannot be ignored. Once these dynamics are understood by the patient he will, of his own accord, accomplish the task in hand. Hence the social worker's task lies merely in making such understanding available to the patient.

5   *Ensuring unimpeded detachment from human relationships*
A fifth aspect of the social worker's terminal crisis work lies in ensuring the patient's unimpeded detachment from relationships in order that he may die with dignity.

As has been discussed in relation to the previous task, suggesting to the terminal patient that he separates himself in preparation for death is likely only to complicate his work. Consequently, the social worker's facilitating response appears to lie in identifying this area of terminal crisis work, remaining alongside the patient while he attempts the task and verbalising any difficulties he may be experiencing in the area. Since difficulties are likely to spring from unresolved life issues the content of this social work task is likely to focus on the past as well as on the future.

Most important, the social worker can ensure the patient's unimpeded detachment from human relationships by working with his relatives in order to enable them to reach an acceptance of their impending loss. This task is undertaken on the assumption that the patient will feel free to detach himself (and so to die peacefully) only once the family accepts the impending separation. The timing is important. Aiding the patient to disengage too early will provoke guilt feelings. Only once acceptance of death is in sight will the patient feel relief as the burden of family relationships is lifted. Thus appropriately timed detachment frees the patient to disengage himself and to die unmolested by relatives. Consequently the social work task of aiding the patient in his disengagement from life, and particularly from former relationships, involves active work both with the patient's relatives and the patient himself.

Case illustration 20: the social worker aids the patient's detachment from relationships

Mrs M, 30 years of age and the mother of two pre-school children, had disseminated carcinoma. The disease had ravaged her body very quickly.

For the past three months she had been seriously ill. Mrs M's mother had travelled a great distance to stay with the family temporarily in order to look after the household and the children. A week before Mrs M died the social worker visited her in her home. Mrs M welcomed her with a lovely, serene smile, but her eyes were penetrating and sad. The interview covered a number of topics, including Mrs M's physical condition, her feelings of sadness and her acceptance of the situation. The worker encouraged Mrs M to express her sadness and difficulties. Then, as though to challenge the worker's power to help her, Mrs M asked what the worker could have arranged, had her mother not been available to look after the house and children.

In posing this question Mrs M appeared to have been preoccupied with detachment. The worker thought that she was asking what facilities existed and what might happen to those whom she was about to 'desert'.

Accordingly, the social worker responded to the naturalness of her concern for those who were to be left behind after she had died. In order to assure Mrs M that her survivors would be adequately cared for, the worker offered some factual information concerning available community facilities. Then, in order to aid Mrs M to continue her work of separating herself from her family, the worker commented that, happily, Mrs M's mother *had* been available and seemed to be of great help to the whole family. This solution to the situation appeared to be a more suitable one than having to call upon community resources. They then discussed the relief which Mrs M experienced at knowing that her family was to be left in good care. She did not need to feel she was deserting them. Mrs M nodded agreement and, with eyes closed, rested her head back, thereby communicating her relief and detachment in word and action.

Mrs M died in hospital a week later.

This illustration shows the importance of timing in the caregiver's terminal crisis work. Had the patient not yet been in the final stage of adjustment to death, discussion of the family's care after Mrs M's death may well have provoked many negative feelings. Here Mrs M *was* ready to discuss family arrangements which excluded her and was relieved to be able to detach herself from them.

In Mrs M's family her relatives were able, without social work intervention, to allow her to disengage herself. Other families might, however, require professional intervention during this period in order to ensure that they do not restrain the patient's disengagement from life.*

6 *Providing a climate in which spiritual issues may be explored*
The ultimate area in which the social worker undertakes terminal crisis work with the patient is that of spiritual preparation for death. A number of social work writers have stressed the need to consider spirit-

* See case illustration 22, Mrs I, whose husband 'recalled' her to life, pp. 91–4.

ual issues when undertaking terminal crisis work (Pearson, 1954, and Player, 1954). Among them, McLaurin (1959) expounds the abiding value of the human spirit, for which social work is committed to care. She suggests that the social worker should view life and death on a continuum. In so doing the worker will help the dying person to live as well as to die.

Controversy reigns within the social work profession concerning the role of religion in therapeutic situations (Tilley, 1962). One view claims that the influence of religion is counterproductive in the counselling process, as it advocates the denial and idealisation of difficulties as a means of coping with them. In addition, the long-accepted mandate that social workers ought not to impose their own beliefs has confused the issue, since it has led many of them to avoid this area of counselling work altogether. Player (1954), however, contends that it is impossible to ignore the spiritual aspects of man's nature. She writes 'in our work with dying patients, even if in no other situation, we as social workers . . . may help people to find the spiritual comfort and healing which alone can really sustain them' (p. 484).

This task is listed here as a social work responsibility for several reasons. Firstly, because it is inappropriate to respond to psychosocial and spiritual elements in the situation as though they were separate. Responding to the total person demands that these tasks be integrated. Secondly, spiritual work is listed within social work's sphere of activities because the *patient* often places it there. It appears that just because the social worker does not represent 'morality', 'the church', 'the conscience', or similar notions attached to the belief in there being a judgement of the person after death, the patient often elects to discuss such topics with her, rather than with his chaplain. It would therefore seem a rejection of the client's concerns not to respond, if that is what he raises.

This is not to say that the social worker has the exclusive role to play in this sphere. On the contrary, she cannot do this work without the support and consultation of the other members of the team and, particularly, the chaplain. It is important however to acknowledge that some role confusion seems to exist in this regard. In the past decade the chaplain has frequently seen his role *vis à vis* dying people in the sphere of counselling and brotherly fellowship, rather than in direct discussion of theological issues (Autton, 1969), while the rest of the team has continued to expect him to fill the latter role. Consequently the patient has sometimes been left without any member of the team who is willing and able to discuss spiritual issues with him. This constitutes an additional reason for the social worker's involvement in this sphere.

As in other areas of terminal crisis work the task of the caregiver lies not in inducing spiritual growth but in responding to it when the patient's natural propulsion towards acceptance encompasses development along a spiritual dimension. The social worker then responds to the emergent faith of the patient, irrespective of denomination. For example, for the Judaeo-Christian world the content of this terminal care task is likely to include, *inter alia*, discussions of the patient's beliefs concerning God, life after death, the soul (or spirit) and the use of prayer. These spiritual issues may be raised during any stage of adjustment to dying.

The caregiver may thus respond to or introduce the topic of spiritual preparation for death as one aspect of dealing with the total person. In so doing, however, she needs to consider the personal views of each patient, she should not labour the point and, most important, as in all caring settings she should not impose her own religious philosophy on her dying patient. Her part is to understand his need to develop along a spiritual dimension while dying and to support, respond to and aid him in this aspect of his preparation for death. As such, it is well to note that the tasks in regard to the patient's spiritual and emotional development are not dissimilar.

On the assumption that there is eternal life, it is important to specify the social work activities which arise out of this aspect of terminal crisis work. In providing a climate in which spiritual issues may be explored, the following tasks may be undertaken: assessing the spiritual strengths of the patient and of his relatives; offering spiritual ideas as resources in the terminal situation; enabling the patient to draw upon these resources, where the practice is foreign or elicits guilt feelings; responding to spiritual issues when the patient raises them; responding to the spiritual implications of issues inherent in the terminal situation (for example, suffering, sickness and/or death); introducing a spiritual perspective to the situation, which the patient may or may not wish to discuss further; and, where appropriate, linking spiritual and psychosocial issues as part of the counselling process.

Case illustration 21: terminal crisis work focusing on spiritual issues

Mr L, a 57-year-old widower, had carcinoma of the bronchus. A year after the discovery of his malignant condition, he was admitted to hospital. Medically, he appeared to be entering the final stage of his illness.

EXTRACTS FROM FOURTH CONTACT WITH MR L (in hospital)

Aim: to aid Mr L in his terminal crisis work

The first portion of the interview had focused upon Mr L's awareness of his condition and had established that he knew that he was dying. His associated feelings had been discussed.

Record

Then Mr L talked of his faith in God, of how he prayed for relief of his pain [1] and how this practice helped him – sometimes [2].

Comment

1 In this statement the worker noted progress in Mr L's adjustment to his situation. In earlier contacts he had simply expected to be cared for; here he *asked* for care, in the form of relief from pain.

2 The worker understood the anger experienced when prayers were not answered.

The worker worded for Mr L how difficult it was to pray when he felt weak and grim: it took real effort. Mr L agreed eagerly, relieved that his effort had been recognised. The worker said that she felt sure that God also understood that prayer required effort, and that he did not exact intense effort from a sick man [3]. Mr L agreed.

3 The worker reinforced Mr L's perception of God as an understanding caring being.

The worker asked Mr L whether he believed in an after-life [4]. He was not sure what she meant.
W: I mean heaven.
Mr L: Yes, I believe in heaven.
W: Well, for your suffering, you may well go to heaven . . . [5].

4 Since Mr L was an extremely passive terminal patient, the worker actively directed this discussion.

5 Since Mr L had mentioned God earlier he gave the worker the opportunity of conferring this 're-ward', at a time when he needed to be rewarded.

Mr L: Yes, I have suffered for a whole year now . . . [6].

6 The reward was seen as appropriate and meaningful.

W: Would that [heaven] make it worthwhile [7]?

7 Since meaningful suffering could combat feelings of hopelessness, the worker enabled Mr L to perceive his suffering as worthwhile, if only in terms of the reward which might be forthcoming.

Mr L nodded, with a wholehearted smile and a little silence, as he contemplated going to heaven.

In this illustration spiritual issues featured in the counselling process, in the following way. Mr L was a patient who had tried to live his whole life as a non-questioning child, obedient to authority; in return, he expected to be rewarded, that is, cared for. For him, heaven constituted a reward offered in recognition of his patient bearing of suffering, pain and a hard life. In the interview the worker had reinforced his pattern of obedience-in-order-to-gain-reward as a style of his living and dying. At the same time she had helped him to preserve his hopefulness by enabling him to perceive a purpose in his situation.

It will be noted that the worker introduced the topic of life after death. It has been suggested that terminal caregivers should help their patients to anticipate life after death (Carlozzi, 1968). Leslie (1960) goes further in suggesting that the worker should not wait for the patient to raise spiritual issues; she should initiate such discussion, especially so with weak, confused and passive patients. Mr L's extreme, lifelong passivity placed him in this category of patients. His long history of non-attendance at any church indicated that this sort of discussion with a social worker was acceptable. Neither he nor his family ever mentioned a priest and, consequently, nor did she.

This illustration also demonstrates how various terminal problem-solving tasks are undertaken parallel to each other. For example, elements of all five stages of dying work are evident in this consultation session with Mr L.

Denial
I'm feeling better.

Isolation
I try not to talk about my illness to my family.

Anger
I've worked hard all my life (but now I nevertheless have to suffer).

Bargaining
If I suffer silently, I'll be cared for.
If I suffer silently, I may go to Heaven.

Depression
I'm down in the dumps.
I'm fit to die.
My body gave up.

Acceptance
I'm pleased to die.
It will have been worth it.

In contrast to Mr L in case illustration 21, Mrs I provides an illustration of a patient with staunch religious beliefs who maintained her faith throughout her terminal illness and died with dignity. A number of caregivers commented after her death that Mrs I had been mature and noble, that her faith had been her obvious support while dying and that caring for her had constituted a salutary experience.

Case illustration 22: adjustment to the terminal situation, motivated by faith

Mrs I, 41 years old, a wife and the mother of two sickly children, had disseminated carcinoma of the ovary. She spent the last nine weeks of her life in hospital, where she died after abdominal obstruction.

In the last three months of Mrs I's terminal illness the social worker held twenty-one consultation sessions with her. It appeared to the worker that in order to master her crisis Mrs I worked consciously and calmly on five problem areas: adjustment to hospitalisation, awareness and concomitant control of her situation, the care of her children, her response to her physical deterioration and spiritual preparation for death. Only when all five areas of concern had been resolved did she feel ready to die.

1 ADJUSTMENT TO HOSPITALISATION

The first issue with which Mrs I concerned herself was that of her hospitalisation. Six weeks before her death she had hoped still to go home for some weekends and perhaps to stay at home for one or two short periods. She planned how she might receive her injections at home while coming to the hospital only for radiotherapy. She felt that there was something to be done at home but waited to be guided as to what it was. As the possibility of abdominal obstruction increased she managed to go home for only one more weekend and then was not permitted to go home again. During the weekend at home she had been very ill and uncomfortable and her family had been worried, but were unable to make her comfortable. As a result she came to accept that she would never go home again. She was relieved to come back to the hospital when feeling so unwell and from then on she knew that she belonged in the hospital.

2 AWARENESS AND CONTROL OF HER SITUATION

A second area of death work in which Mrs I was engaged was that of her awareness of her condition. Throughout her illness Mrs I was aware and able to talk of her imminent death. She was alert, participated in her own care and was upset with herself on days when she was sleepy throughout the day (even though, intellectually, she knew that her medication had had some sedative effect). It became clear that one of the issues that concerned Mrs I was that of control. She had as her unspoken aim that of remaining in control of herself, of the expression of her emotions and of her whole situation. Drowsiness made control difficult so that she said she 'felt so stupid' when she was less alert and that she felt better and happier the next day when she was more alert again.

Two weeks before her death Mrs I acknowledged that she was ready to die, but said that she did not feel it was quite her time yet. As her condition worsened physically Mrs I engaged in assessing her readiness to die and how much time she still had on earth. Her awareness remained complete; the only uncertainty lay in the question: 'How long?' To answer this question, Mrs I used her physical condition as her guide. For example, she could not understand how she could sip clear water and moments later bring up awful, discoloured fluid. She did not realise that her abdomen was a cancerous mass, and was momentarily frightened at the thought of how decayed her body had become. After another patient in the ward had died whom Mrs I had earlier heard gasping for breath, she commented to the social worker that she was not nearly dead yet, 'because I still have a lot of breath. I heard, a person must have little breath before you die.' Mrs I then pondered upon the causes and course of dying and told the social worker of neighbours who had been killed in a motor accident: 'You don't even need to be sick to die.'

After living through a week in which the staff had thought she would die, Mrs I discussed her survival with the social worker. They had previously talked of borrowed time and Mrs I had said that she regarded such time as a blessing. She had not been aware, during that critical week, that her physical condition had been so grave and had not felt that death was at hand. Consequently, she questioned the event in surprise and when the social worker confirmed that death had indeed been very close she found the information meaningful. She tried to piece together other things that had been said to her during that period in an attempt to make sense of them. She mused on dying and death for quite a while, trying, in retrospect, to work out what death would be like if she had been so near it already and had not realised it. She tried to work out why she had survived that episode. What was God's plan now? Was she not ready yet? How should she use the time still left to her?

3   THE CARE OF HER CHILDREN

A third area of Mrs I's dying work concerned her relationship with her family. At first she expressed concern about the care of her two sickly children and particularly wished to discuss the facts of life with her early-adolescent daughter. 'After all, it is still a mother's task', she commented. Mrs I accomplished this task during her last weekend at home. Thereafter she said relatively little about her family until she was ready to disengage from them. At that point Mrs I's protection of and concern for her family were evident, among other ways, in her request that the social worker should contact them. At the same time, however, she cautioned the social worker to talk kindly and to beware lest the truth of the situation upset them.

One day Mrs I said that she felt that her parents were with her in spirit, to help her, and that she was especially sure that her mother was with her. When the social worker asked her how she knew, she answered, 'You can just feel it'. She was comforted by the thought that she might in the same way be able to continue her help and guidance to her children once she was dead.

After not discussing the topic for some time the worker referred to Mrs I's concern regarding her children and realised that the reason for her silence on this issue resulted from her resolution of the problem. Mrs I told the worker calmly that she no longer wondered what would happen to them, as she knew that God would care for them when she was gone. Mrs I was thus fairly easily able to let go of her earthly ties and responsibilities, because by then she had come to know that she was confidently giving them over into God's care.

4   RESPONSE TO PHYSICAL DETERIORATION

A fourth area of terminal crisis work which Mrs I managed successfully related to her response to her physical deterioration. She endured painful procedures bravely but was nevertheless able to admit how unpleasant these were and indicated when she could tolerate no more. For example, three litres of abdominal fluid were tapped over six days during which she hardly complained, because she was comforted by the thought that 'Jesus had to go through more'. On the sixth day she realistically acknowledged depression and said that she had had enough.

Mrs I was unable to keep food down and grew painfully thin. She was constantly uncomfortable. She vomited often, but always managed on her own to use the kidney bowl and not to foul herself or her bed. She managed this so unobtrusively that other patients in the ward hardly noticed that she had been sick.

As Mrs I grew more and more uncomfortable she acknowledged that no one could help her any more. This realisation appeared to be the most difficult aspect of all to bear. She longed for the relief of death.

5   SPIRITUAL PREPARATION FOR DEATH

Throughout her life Mrs I had been a devout churchgoer, with firm faith. She knew from the onset that she had cancer. She knew what the implications were and talked freely of these issues to the social worker. On first hearing her diagnosis, she had felt alone, sad and discouraged, but that had lasted only 'while I fought with my maker'. Her main concern was to work out how much time she had left and how God wanted her to use it. Initially she felt that she would regain some strength, as she still had work to do. When questioned by the social worker as to what she hoped to do, she talked of spending the rest of her life in the service of God. They discussed how difficult it was at times to 'wait on the Lord' apparently doing nothing, but serving him still.

Mrs I perceived death essentially in spiritual terms: 'I'll open my eyes in Jesus Christ; it's the beginning, not the end.' This perspective did not, however, lead to denial or idealisation of the situation; on the contrary, Mrs I remained realistic in coping with and talking of her illness.

Throughout the terminal situation Mrs I's faith was evident as a recurrent area of dying work. She had a well-used bible at her bedside and often talked of things she had read. She prayed for other patients as well as for herself and accepted the prayers of others graciously, saying with surprise, 'A person never knows when he needs the prayers of others more than his own'. Each of the issues that she had worked on had been resolved with the aid of prayer, which she gratefully acknowledged after her petitions had been answered. She experienced little isolation, because she was sure of the presence of God. Her firm belief in an after life was an apparent source of strength to her. She looked forward to heaven, and pondered earnestly on whether she needed to worry about going to hell. At length, she thought not. Mrs I had two spirit-experiences of dying before she actually died. The first occurred three weeks before death. She experienced that she was dying: she felt she was far away and going further, but her husband pulled her back by calling her and shaking her body. Her mother had been there to greet her. She had been calm and unafraid. On her 'return', her reaction was the sad realisation of 'Oh, I'm still here'.

Mrs I's second spirit experience of dying occurred three days before her death. In the early hours of a long night, she had felt, somehow, that she was dying and had felt frightened. She had to call a staff member in order not to be alone . . . and then she remembered to hold Jesus's hand and felt calmer. When she awoke, she felt heartsore at having disappointed Jesus by feeling fear. By the morning, she was calmer again, except for feeling guilty about the episode.

The social worker discussed these feelings with her, helping her to verbalise and accept them as natural rather than as weakness, as Mrs I was perceiving them. She acknowledged that it was the devil that had made her frightened and said how unready she felt to fight him while in her present weakened state. She knew, however, that she had to repel his attack. She was helped to express how unfair she felt it was to be attacked while she was 'down'. The worker then reminded her of the protection that was at her disposal, and Mrs I responded that she knew that Jesus was with her.

On the day of her death, Mrs I became confused and dozed a good deal. Her husband remained with her until she died. A few hours before she died, she awoke and expressed her impatience to be relieved by asking 'Why can't I go?' and dozed without an answer. Her last words, a little later, were: 'My little time is up. I'm going to my Lord.'

COMMENT

It thus became apparent that Mrs I prepared for death by working on herself, trying to estimate what the unknown event might demand of her and taking pains to remain cheerful and uncomplaining while dying. Her particular strength lay in an ability to acknowledge her difficulties and her negative feelings (for example, fear, depression and guilt). While she did not inhibit or deny these emotions, she did control their expression. For example, she tried not to let her distress upset other patients in the ward and she expressed her depression to the social worker while presenting a more cheerful exterior to her relatives.

Mrs I's realistic yet self-controlled conduct thus appeared to constitute her dignity, and earned her the respect, affection and care of all around her.

Mrs I demonstrates that the faith of the terminal patient can play a major facilitative role in adjustment to death, and that faith is one part of the whole person which overlaps with feelings and attitudes to life. The illustration is presented in such detail because it answers the challenge that religion advocates the denial and idealisation of life's pain and conflicts. On the contrary, Mrs I's dying bears out the claim made in Chapter 3 that religious faith does not obviate the conflicts of life – or death – but can provide the people concerned with the strength to face and resolve them. Terminal crisis work with Mrs I would thus have been incomplete had spiritual issues not featured prominently.

TERMINAL CRISIS WORK WITH THE FAMILY

So far we have discussed terminal crisis work as work with the dying person directly. It may of course also include work with his relatives as well. Indeed, work with the family of the patient is vital if we are to ensure effective work in terminal care. Here the caregiver responds both to the patient and also to the family's efforts to resolve the crisis inherent in the terminal situation. In addition, since the patient's family may form part of the treatment team where, say, one close relative, with the support and guidance of the rest of the team, becomes the primary caregiver, that relative qualifies for professional help, both in his own right and on the patient's behalf.

The content of terminal crisis work with relatives includes topics similar to those discussed with the patient. It may cover the various tasks which are involved in the resolution of the terminal crisis, with some of which the family is already likely to be engaged. These issues are dealt with both in an effort to facilitate the patient's mastery of the crisis and from the perspective of the relatives themselves. Again, in practice this counselling involves helping the family to face death by helping them to face life. Rather than simply marking time while they await the death, they can be helped to use this preparatory period creatively (Daniel, 1973).

As the relatives progress through the various psychosocial stages towards acceptance of the patient's death, their adjustment may not keep pace with that of the patient (Kübler-Ross, 1970a). Consequently the social worker needs to respond to each stage of their adjustment in order to facilitate their achievement of acceptance and at the same time synchronise reactions, so that the patient and his relatives reach acceptance of the situation at approximately the same time. Terminal crisis work with the relatives of the patient also concentrates, after the death, on the process of mourning (Daniel, 1973).

While the patient is dying family members need particular help in dealing with their feelings of guilt and regret in relation to the patient. In this connection Daniel (1973) writes: 'The social worker helps the family to try to hold a balance between the continuing living events of daily life, and the preparation for the losing of the person who is going to die.' Pilsecker (1975) stresses that the social worker should ensure that neither the patient nor his family is engaged in game-playing regarding the impending death. It is therefore important for her to involve the family in communications regarding the patient's awareness of his condition. In this way the various participants in the situation are kept abreast of the progress of the others and deception, prevarications and half-truths are obviated. The family is freed to make optimal use of the shortened time still available to it. The most typical work with families of the dying person concerns this area of awareness and consequent communication within the family. Achieving open communication avoids both the patient's intense isolation and the family's regrets of deception and game-playing after the patient has died.

Perhaps it is fair to alert the reader to the difficulties involved in this sort of work with the relatives of a dying person. It has been my experience on many occasions that family members experience very mixed feelings regarding the efforts of an outside caregiver. On the one hand there is relief at the added help that is forthcoming to their difficult situation. An outsider brings perspective, balance, understanding, distractions, collusion (sometimes) to any game-playing that may be in progress, and unquestioned support for the relatives.

But at the same time an outsider – especially if she is a professional caregiver – brings skill in responding to the patient. Such contact with the dying person may be experienced by his relatives as a reproach to their own feelings of inadequacy and helplessness and so increases their feelings of guilt. The skills of the caregiver may be envied, as a result of which her presence is resented and devalued. The fact that the patient may benefit from her visit, or requests to see her again, only reinforces the whole situation. Hence relatives of the dying person may often be hostile to an outside caregiver and may compete with her in their care of the patient, or make it difficult for her to tend the patient at all.

It may be difficult for the caregiver to remind herself not to take such rebuffs personally. Part of such hostility may be an expression of the family's anger, directed towards the caregiver as a representative of the medical service which is failing to cure their loved one. Another part of that anger may be likened to the abusing mother who resents professional intervention as it highlights her inadequate mothering. Such anger is appropriate: we need constantly to remind ourselves that relatives have the first claim to the care of the dying person. Any 'help' which is intrusive, uncaringly critical of the efforts of relatives or insensitive to their right to be there, deserves to be resented and barred from further intrusion. It is therefore essential whenever possible to see our role *vis à vis* the family as one of helping *them* to tend their loved one, rather than one in which we take over and displace them from their natural, rightful place in the team.

Case illustration 23: terminal crisis work with a relative of a patient

MRS D'S SITUATION

Mrs D, 41 years old, wife and mother of a young son, had disseminated carcinoma. The worker had seen Mrs D thirteen times in six months. She had been admitted to hospital six weeks prior to this interview on account of the spread of the carcinoma. She was receiving radiotherapy and chemotherapy and was experiencing unpleasant side effects from both treatment methods.

CIRCUMSTANCES OF EXTENDING THE SOCIAL WORK   SERVICE
TO MRS D'S HUSBAND

Mrs D has been told that her disease had continued its spread. She had shared this information with her husband and was concerned on account of his distress. Since then five weeks had elapsed during which time Mrs D had received hospitalised treatment during the week and gone home at weekends. She was weaker, often in pain, but still wanted to do more at home than she could and felt guilty about her debility. As a result she often responded by being 'bitchy' to her husband. She returned to the hospital feeling worse on account of her uselessness at home.

At the worker's suggestion Mrs D agreed that the worker should contact her husband and arrange an interview. Mrs D asked the worker to explain why she was so 'bitchy' to him, and to let him know that she was troubled by the awful weekend that they had just spent together. Mrs D insisted that the worker should not let her husband know that she (Mrs D) was aware that the worker was contacting her husband. The worker agreed in order that Mrs D should not feel more threatened than was necessary. She planned instead to discuss the issue of open communication between husband and wife when next she saw Mrs D. She estimated that if she were to refuse Mrs D's stipulation the request might be withdrawn altogether. Therefore, wanting also to offer support to Mr D, the worker accepted the condition imposed by the patient.

She did not at that stage discuss the issue of collusion with Mrs D, who might have wondered about the social worker's willingness to see one member of the family at the instigation of another.

INITIAL INTERVIEW WITH MR D (at the hospital)

Aim of the interview

The aims of the interview were to establish contact with Mr D; to assess the family's situation and their need of social work aid in their own right; to support Mr D in relation to his wife's experience; to discuss practical aspects of the situation; and to inform him of the research project.

Client: Mr D

Mr D appeared to be a sensitive, gentle person, who talked freely, frankly and with feeling. He was near to tears throughout the session. The worker helped him to contain himself and recognise that he was coping with his situation. At the same time she remained sympathetic to the difficulties of his position.

On reflection the social worker realised that throughout the interview she had identified far more with Mrs D, her patient, than with the interviewee, the patient's husband. Theoretically she had aimed to offer Mr D support and understanding of his difficulties but in fact she had allowed him only limited opportunities to ventilate his feelings. There were two reasons for this:

(a) since the interview took place just prior to hospital visiting time the worker estimated that it would not be helpful to enable Mr D to ventilate too freely as he was likely to break down and would still have to face his wife immediately afterwards;

(b) the focus of the social worker's service to the family centred on Mrs D, the terminal patient. She was the worker's primary patient. It thus became very difficult for the worker to perceive the situation simultaneously in terms of the fears, fantasies and feelings of Mrs D and other members of the family as well.

Consequently, the worker did not respond to all the feelings which Mr D was experiencing at that time. She was, however, able to hold the feelings which he brought to the meeting even though they were not all explicitly clarified.

Record	*Comment*
Mr D appeared surprised to hear that his wife had had discussions with the worker over the past months. He asked her how often she had seen his wife [1]. She answered by stressing her availability to them both and said that she understood what a difficult time it was for all of them, and that she therefore wanted to be used in any way that they might find useful. Mr D accepted this interpretation of the worker's role and began to use the interview [2].	1 The worker understood that the threat of being excluded from the social worker's relationship with his wife might prevent Mr D from making use of the social work service. It was understandable that he felt possessive of his now short-lived relationship with his wife and that he felt threatened by the worker's intrusion into their lives. In an effort to overcome this possible barrier she therefore stressed her understanding of his situation and her availability to them both. At this point Mr D's feelings of exclusion could, perhaps, have been focused upon.
	2 Despite the potentially threatening beginning, something positive must have been communicated be-

Record

Comment

cause Mr D was able to make maximum use of this interview. He immediately asked for advice and did not resist the worker's attempts to enable him to look for some answers and explanations for himself. Perhaps his own disequilibrium, at a time of situational crisis in his life, made him amenable to the help offered. The social work intervention thus appeared to have been timely.

He asked how much he should say to his wife concerning her terminal situation and told the worker that at present he was playing it by ear one day at a time, taking his cues from her. The worker supported him in this approach, clarifying that he was focusing on his wife's needs and moods, and that while this attitude was very helpful to her, it was probably difficult for him to maintain.

Mr D asked the worker whether he should begin to build a flatlet on to their home, as Mrs D had recently suggested. He had planned that he and his son could live in the flatlet, while the house could be let to a good friend of theirs.

Mrs D had previously told the worker of this scheme [3]. She had also anticipated that her husband might eventually marry this friend. She had said that she would not mind this arrangement as she loved the two of them, her husband and friend, very dearly and would be pleased if they could make each other happy.

3 Mrs D's attempts for the future seemed to indicate her need to control her situation. This plan might also be interpreted as a wish to perpetuate herself. At the same time, planning for her family's future offered a way of easing her guilt feelings concerning her inability to cope with present responsibilities.

The worker responded by helping Mr D to understand what his wife was doing, and why. She suggested that Mrs D was feeling guilty on account of not being able to maintain her wifely and motherly respon-

Record

sibilities, and was absolving herself of these duties by making 'suitable' arrangements for her family for the future. Thereafter, knowing that things were being taken care of, she could detach herself. Mr D wondered, then, whether he should act on her suggestions. The worker advised that he should comply only if these plans suited *him* too. Perhaps he could wait to see if his wife raised the issue again, to gauge how strongly she felt about it.

The worker suggested that Mr D might consider how his wife would be affected [4] if he did carry out her plans and helped him to see that she might feel rejected if he already began to plan and think about the future while she was still alive. He accepted this caution.

The worker then, indiscreetly [5] disclosed to Mr D that his wife had already anticipated that he might eventually marry his friend. She told Mr D that Mrs D would support this decision, as it would bring happiness to the two people whom she had loved very dearly in life. Mr D's eyes brimmed at this news. After a short silence, the worker helped him to express how difficult the present situation was for himself, his wife and their child.

Comment

4 The worker overidentified with Mrs D's position, to a point of exclusion of Mr D's feelings on the matter.

5 The worker was ambivalent in her motivation for telling Mr D that his wife had anticipated his remarriage. She wished to see, on Mrs D's behalf, if this idea was at all feasible to her husband. She was also partly motivated to tell him of Mrs D's idea because if the marriage ever came to pass it might be helpful to him to know that she was happy about it too.

The worker was aware of disclosing something from her relationship with a patient to another person (without the prior consent of the patient). More appropriately, she should have obtained permission to tell her husband, or supported Mrs D's own efforts to discuss this issue with her husband.

The disclosure, which stemmed partly from the worker's inability to hold so much impending tragedy, unhelpfully made Mr D look towards the future, instead of allowing him to ventilate his

Record

In response to the worker's questioning Mr D talked about his management of his son and home.

The worker listened, showed understanding of the practical difficulties of the situation and tried to show Mr D that he *was* managing to cope with a great deal, despite the emotional strain of his situation.

The worker noted that this interview constituted Mr D's first contact with a representative of the hospital staff, and discussed how they might keep in touch in the future.

Mr D talked of his wife [6], describing her both when she was in pain and when she was feeling cheerful. He acknowledged how hard she was trying – successfully – to be bright, cheerful and content. Her mood depended on her pain. This remark gave the worker an opportunity of explaining Mrs D's apparent rudeness, guilt and ambivalence. They discussed Mrs D's attempts to work out what was going on in her life and her wish, as in the past, to be strong and able to 'take it'. The worker helped Mr D to understand Mrs D's need to be in control of some things in her situation, while at the same time feeling relief at being able to let go of responsibilities. As a result of what was said Mr D seemed to understand his wife's position better. The worker also commented on Mrs D's strengths [7] and expressed her admiration of Mrs D's preparedness to work on all the problem areas in her situation.

Comment

present anguish and anticipated loss.

6 It seemed that once Mr D's own situation had received some attention, support and an offer of continuing help in the future, he was able again to focus on what his wife was experiencing, in an effort to help her.

7 Although the worker might more helpfully have focused on Mr D's feelings regarding the difficulty of the situation, he seemed encouraged by the worker's observation of the strengths which both he and Mrs D possessed. Listing Mrs D's strength realistically appeared to have the effect of relieving Mr

Record

Towards the end of the interview, the worker thanked Mr D [8] and told him how helpful it had been to talk to him. In return, Mr D thanked the worker and then wondered whether he should tell his wife that he had seen her. She asked what he felt like doing. He wasn't sure. The worker wondered whether he wanted to start a deception at this stage [9] after having come so far without it. Mr D supposed not. He was very grateful to the worker. She agreed to keep in touch with him.

Comment

D of part of his burden. He was reassured that she could cope with her situation, and he could manage his part in the crisis.

The social worker had conveyed support and encouragement to Mr D. Unwittingly she might however have set a standard that was too high for Mr D to maintain. This act could have led to anger and consequently to resistance in using social work aid in the future.

8 The worker was aware of the mutuality of the helping relationship, both with patients and their relatives. At a time of crisis, potential dependence and guilt about his helplessness, the worker felt it was helpful to acknowledge Mr D's ability to be of assistance to her.
9 The worker imposed her view concerning deception.

EVALUATION

Mr D's gratitude was marked. The worker assessed that he was responding not only to the social worker's help in that particular interview but to the fact that, at last, the hospital was talking to him and treating him as a person.

Mr D appeared to be contained, in touch with his feelings, and amenable to social work help. He made good use of this interview and was able to receive the worker's support. He felt relief as a result of being able to share his difficulties and it was helpful to him that the worker could contain and acknowledge some of his feelings and emotions. Most of the focus of the interview rested on his wife's feelings, rather than on Mr D's own. Nevertheless, the worker felt that he had been encouraged, and that he had benefited from the time which they had spent together.

The worker was favourably impressed by Mr D's sincerity, his wish to help his wife, his frank discussion and his ability to put his own feelings in the background and to do instead what was best for Mrs D. Mr D appeared to be mastering a difficult situation.

FUTURE PLANS

Continue to support and help both Mr and Mrs D to work toward adjustment of their respective crises. If Mr D does not approach the worker, she should contact him again. Encourage Mr and Mrs D to share their feelings with each other and to share their contact with the worker.

This illustration shows that terminal crisis work with the relative of the patient focuses its help both on the relative *per se* and on the relative in his role as caregiver to the patient. As with terminal crisis work with the patient, work with his relatives involves some tasks that are special to the terminal situation. They are:

7 facilitating the patient/family's decision with regard to the extraordinary prolongation of life;
8 aiding bereaved relatives with their grief work.

7 *Facilitating the patient/family's decision with regard to the extradordinary prolongation of life*

Terminal crisis work may also sometimes include facilitating decisions regarding resuscitation and life-prolonging procedures. Where this task applies, it requires negotiation with all the parties involved in the situation: patient, relatives and other members of the team, together and separately, as each party needs to take the points of view of the others into consideration. Obviously it can only be undertaken within the existing laws regarding euthanasia.

There are some situations in which such resuscitative decisions are appropriately made by the medical team, without consultation with the patient or his family. There are other situations in which it is crucial that the views of the patient and his relatives are taken into account. But since this practice is relatively unfamiliar within the medical model, the social worker has important work to do to ensure that the views of the patient and his family are given a fair hearing.

This task involves creating a climate of trust in which honest views can be expressed with regard to the patient's desire to continue living or not. Because the patient's wish to die may be perceived by relatives as the ultimate rejection, and vice versa, this issue requires delicate timing, skill and discretion. The caregiver needs to assess very accurately what the patient and relatives are saying, feeling and meaning. The decision, like that of whether to 'tell' or not, will be based in part on the worker's assessment of their past experiences of stress, decision-making and patterns of coping – particularly in situations involving separation, loss and dependence. Where the patient and family have reached their decisions separately, the social worker may act as catalyst in bringing them together to face each other with their decisions, take leave of each other, complete some unfinished business, use the time as fully as they wish and/or to plan for the future.

8 *Aiding bereaved relatives with their grief work*
Terminal crisis work with the relatives of the patient also includes, after the death, aiding them with their process of mourning (Daniel, 1973). At such time those families who believe that life continues after death will take comfort in the knowledge that they will eventually be reunited with their loved one. Nevertheless the present loss is grave and requires considerable grief work before the death of the patient can be adjusted to.

The social worker's task here is to ensure that the survivors do in fact do their grief work, both as a means of adjustment to the present situation and as a means of preventing psychological disturbance in the future. Helping them to cope with this loss will equip them to cope with many other life crises and future tasks, and particularly those involving loss. Facilitating grief work requires that the social worker helps the relatives to experience, express and then contain their feelings of sadness and hostility. Again, her interventions respond to what the survivors are experiencing or to the mourning work they are doing for themselves. Skill is required here to mention the unmentionable and, often, to violate social and cultural taboos in order to do so. Unless the worker can comfortably talk of the deceased person, dying, death and loss, and help the survivors to do so too, she will not be able to help them to liberate themselves from their relationships with the deceased person and equip themselves for life without him. If she can facilitate grief work they will be able to take something positive from this experience for use in their own lives and in their future relationship with others.

SOCIAL GROUP WORK

For the sake of completeness social group work also merits some mention, although on the whole its application to the field of terminal care is no different from its practice in other settings. The use of groups as a medium of helping bereaved people has been well documented (Lindemann, 1944; Snelling, 1966; Schoenberg *et al.*, 1970; Parkes, 1972; McCollum and Schwartz, 1972; Daniel, 1973). But because relatives of a terminal patient often experience similar situations while the patient is still alive, Knapp and Hansen (1973) and Pilsecker (1975) have also stressed the particular value of helping such people while they are preparing for a loss, through the use of a group. Some concern has been expressed regarding terminal crisis work with more than one person at a time. But groups have nevertheless been recommended as one vital medium for offering terminal crisis counselling both to the dying person and his family members. Here the social worker can offer several people an opportunity of sharing feelings and experiences, combating their isolation and overcoming their feelings of impotence and helplessness, by helping others in a similar situation to their own (Goldberg, 1973; Knapp and Hansen, 1973; and Pilsecker, 1975).

Several natural elements in any group provide safeguards to the social worker who is apprehensive of social group work with dying persons or their relatives. She need not fear that the intense individual emotions once merged will reach uncontainable proportions, since it is likely that different group members will be at different stages of their dying work from week to week, so that some will usually be in a position to balance and comfort the anguish of others. In other words the rich resources of other people are available to the worker, thus lightening her load. Another safeguard to terminal crisis work in a group lies in the natural balance that is likely to emerge between discussion of strong emotional issues around dying and more superficial practical difficulties of living, and how they may be overcome. And since the group will set its own pace the worker can be assured that she does not hold the entire responsibility for maintaining this balance herself.

ENVIRONMENTAL MANAGEMENT

A third social work function in the category of work rendered directly to the patient and his family is environmental management. Like terminal crisis work, environmental management aims to facilitate the patient's resolution of his terminal crisis but, unlike the former, it accomplishes its goal by providing practical aid for the patient and his family.

Early social work writings have emphasised the practical responsibilities of the social worker in terminal care (Cockerill, 1937). More recently however the non-material aspects of social work have been given priority (Pearson, 1954; Player, 1954; Birley, 1960· Goldstein, 1973; Chambers, 1974; Weisberg, 1974; and Pilsecker, 1975). For example, Birley points out that financial matters generally become a subsidiary problem during the terminal stage of illness. While this statement may well apply to the patient, financial matters sometimes constitute a major concern for the family, especially if the illness is a protracted one.

When the social worker does engage in environmental management in terminal care she needs to be careful to allow the dying patient as much independent adult action as he is capable of. Weisman (1972a) cautions that the dying person should be permitted to make his own decisions for as long as he possibly can. At the same time, however, the social worker needs to enable him to accept dependence on others.

Environmental management as applied to terminal care encompasses the tasks of determining the need for and appropriateness of resources for terminal care, forming new informal systems for the terminal patient (for example, a befriending service) and locating resources for the terminal patient (for example, local volunteers). Some of these environmental tasks are likely to be shared with other team members, for example, providing knowledge and skills to people who are acting as resources (for example, family caregivers); preparing the terminal patient to use a resource (for example, chemotherapy treatment); helping him use it effectively; and monitoring and supervising the use of the resource (for example, a domiciliary care and support programme). The reader is again reminded that the listing of these environmental tasks as the work of the social worker is not meant to imply that she is the most important caregiver.

All of these tasks apply to environmental management and to the dispensing of material resources in any field. (Pincus and Minahan, 1973). In terminal care, however, I believe that one more specific environmental task may need to be incorporated. Again it is a task shared by doctor, nurse and social worker: planning where terminal care can best be offered.

Planning where terminal care can best be offered
In communities which have no specific terminal care institutions the decision as to where terminal care can best be offered is debated in terms of care either at home or in hospital. Since general hospital policy often does not favour the accommodation of patients with an incurable disease, relatively few terminal patients are cared for in hospitals.

This statement is not to be confused with Sudnow's (1967) observation that in contemporary times more people die in hospitals than has been the case in former years. Many patients however are admitted to hospital only when already unconscious, just prior to death. Consequently, although they *die* in hospital, the bulk of their care has been managed at home, or in a cycle of care at home, hospital, then home and hospital again.

The social worker's task thus lies in helping the terminal patient/ family to assess the advantages and disadvantages of care at home or in hospital (or nursing home); helping them to make realistic decisions with regard to the patient's care; where necessary, arranging practical support for their execution of their plan (for example, financial aid, transport, or domiciliary services); and guiding them to modify plans and arrangements in accordance with the patient's changing medical situation.

Chapter 7

WORKING WITH SIGNIFICANT OTHERS

We have so far discussed the work that the social worker does directly with the patient and his family. But, as Pincus and Minahan's (1973) model suggests, it is not enough to work only with the patient and family. Other significant people in the environment also need to be considered in order to offer an effective service, that is, to ensure that their attitudes, approach and feelings enhance rather than hamper the patient's dying. We therefore need to focus some attention on the inter- action between the terminal patient and his environment and on our collaboration with our colleagues for his benefit.

Pincus and Minahan (1973) term the social work function referred to here as facilitating interaction with and within resource systems. The skill areas required to execute these functions, in any setting, include forming, maintaining and co-ordinating action systems (or teams) and exercising influence. Applying these concepts to terminal care, I have termed the social work functions which emerge: interpretive work be- tween social work and the health disciplines, community work; and educating for terminal care.

INTERPRETIVE WORK BETWEEN SOCIAL WORK AND THE HEALTH DISCIPLINES

Where patients are treated in a multidisciplinary setting (for example, a hospital) if total patient care is to be effective it demands co-operative and co-ordinated efforts on the part of all the team members. Where the team does not function efficiently each worker, in the interests of optimal patient care, bears the responsibility of ensuring its effective operation.

A number of social work writers have motivated social work efforts towards effective interpretive work between social work and the health disciplines, especially in terminal care work. For example, Lang and Oppenheimer (1968) have found that it is possible for consistent social work input to influence the treatment milieu, thereby easing the stress of fatal illness in children. Foster (1965) reports similar observations from her work with adults with an incurable disease. And Goldstein (1973) has also stressed that the patient's dying may be eased or hindered by his impinging environment. Thus the call for interpretive work seems to be unanimous.

The content of interpretive work does not differ substantively from one medical setting to another. In terminal care it usually includes discussion on the nature of the terminal crisis, each patient's particular problem areas in the situation, the implications thereof for patient care and, sometimes, the effects of this work on the caregivers. In addition, Foster (1965) stresses that it includes some examination of the effect of existing communication patterns on the overall treatment programme. It also demands that consideration be given to the specificity, compatibility and efficacy of the roles of staff, patient and relatives. Finally, it needs to take cognisance of Sudnow's (1967) observations of the institutionalisation of death and its implications for patient care.

Case illustration 24: interpretive work between the social worker and a health professional (ward sister)

A ward sister was informed that one of her terminal patients appeared to be depressed. Her comment to the social worker was: 'I'm not happy about Mrs X. She's weepy. I don't want any depressed patients in my ward.' The social worker responded by reinterpreting the situation. She suggested that the patient's depression was understandable and that it constituted a normal, appropriate response to her situation. The social worker then helped the ward sister to consider how such terminal depression might best be handled, both in Mrs X's case and in general. Recognising the anxiety behind the sister's remarks, the social worker acknowledged how one depressed patient could easily affect the atmosphere of the whole ward and reflected that perhaps the ward sister perceived the atmosphere in her ward as a reflection of her management of it. If so, perhaps she held herself responsible for 'weepy' patients in her ward and felt that they represented her failure to nurse them cheerfully.

The ward sister acknowledged that she did perceive depressed patients in this light. The social worker could then focus on the difficulty of the ward sister's position, since many of her (terminal) patients were not cheerful.

Together they pursued some of the sister's feelings concerning terminal care work. She told the social worker of events leading to the death of one of her family members, and how that situation had been handled. The worker allowed her to re-experience some of the pain of that death and then interpreted the ward sister's action: was she not responding to the present situation as she had to a personal experience of dying? How appropriate was that reaction, for herself or her patients?

After some discussion the social worker ended this informal interchange by stressing the appropriateness of some of the terminal reactions which had been mentioned; and she encouraged the ward sister to permit her patients to express these (normal) feelings.

This illustration demonstrates the social worker's interpretive response to a contact with a colleague. It is not my intention here to compare non-social work colleagues with the social worker who, in this example, appears to be competent and understanding. The context in which this incident occurred was one of a social worker pioneering terminal care in a hospital setting in which few colleagues, at that time, had developed terminal care skills. Happily this situation is today somewhat altered.

The interchange was effective on two counts. The caregivers had an already established relationship on which to build further co-operation; and since trust existed between the two colleagues, the ward sister was not threatened by the social worker's ideas. The illustration also shows that interpretive work rests upon the assumption that greater insight into the nature of the terminal crisis facilitates the management of the situation. Thus this social work function frequently includes a repetition of some theoretical considerations involved in terminal crisis work.

As in other fields of social work, the art of interpretive work in terminal care lies in conveying information and attitudes to members of other professions without appearing to criticise their perspective on the situation, without telling colleagues what to do and without posing a personal threat in other members of the team. In terminal care work, however, prevailing attitudes and fears of dying and death and hence whole systems of denial (Menzies, 1970) often complicate the task. Therefore if it is preceded by building relationships of trust between the members of the team – for which there is no easy formula – better teamwork is likely to result. In some cases the social worker initiates such discussions, particularly with staff members who are new to terminal care work and who have hesitated to express their feelings about it. Irrespective of who introduces these discussions the social workers can use such opportunities expressly to facilitate the work of the team. Interpretive work may occur through any of the following channels:

(i)   spontaneous, informal discussions, for example, the discussion of special cases as difficulties arise;
(ii) regular, formal contacts, for example, case conferences, ward rounds, and medical records available to different members of the team;
(iii) written communications, for example, letters and reports;
(iv) strategies for innovation or change, for example, research and demonstration projects.

The form this work takes is less important than the fact that some interpretive work does take place, because 'Frequent confrontations between members of various disciplines and specialities . . . almost certainly will raise the standards of all levels of professional competence' (Weisman and Kastenbaum, 1968, p. 45).

Pincus and Minahan (1973, pp. 20–6) list the many techniques and tasks involved in interpretive work in any setting and suggest the scope of such work. Practitioners who are struggling in this area of their service are referred to their work. They may be helped to identify and analyse where their problems lie and what can be done to improve the situation. It is not intended to imply that any one social worker can or should carry out all these tasks. In addition to the interpretive work mentioned so far I have chosen to highlight six tasks which require particular attention in terminal care work although they apply in many other multidisciplinary settings as well. They are:

(1) initiating open communication for terminal care work;
(2) aiding the caregiving team to decide in which awareness context each terminal patient should be cared for;
(3) decoding the patient's behaviour;
(4) ensuring the designation of a primary caregiver;
(5) focusing on the feelings which colleagues experience in relation to their work;
(6) guiding colleagues in the selection and referral of terminal patients for social work intervention.

(1) *Initiating open communication for terminal care work*

One prerequisite for total patient care is open communication between the patient and the team. Since this is unlikely to occur automatically, the social worker is in a good position to ensure that it does happen. There are several reasons why open awareness contexts need to be safeguarded. Given the choice, many doctors would avoid open discussion of death and dying (Lasagna, 1969 and Cramond, 1970). At the same time many patients know that they are dying and wish to talk about it (ibid). Some catalytic work is therefore necessary to bring these two parties together in discussion.

In addition, initiating open communication lessens the patient's isolation which, as we have already seen, is severe. The social worker's task lies in creating the kind of caring environment in which communication can flow freely back and forth, up and down. In this way the ideal of enabling the patient to tell his caregivers what he knows, instead of vice versa, can occur. A final reason for initiating open awareness contexts in terminal care work is that an informed patient (or relative) who understands the illness and the treatment becomes an invaluable collaborator in the management of the situation.

The social worker can thus ensure open communication in the situation both by initiating it and by maintaining it once established. There is no easy formula as to how to execute this task. Foster's (1965) near classic article offers us one useful giude by stressing the social worker's role as mediator and advocate of the dying patient's rights. Where sound relationships exist between the various members of the care-giving team, the confronting and challenging roles required of her in this task are likely to be more acceptable to her colleagues.

(2) *Aiding the caregiving team to decide in which awareness context each terminal patient should be cared for*

As has already been mentioned the question 'Should the doctor tell?' has been much debated (Kelly and Freisen, 1950; Hinton, 1968b; Saunders, 1976; and others). In many cases the answer has been agreed upon: each case should be judged on its own merits. Consequently the caregiving team has to decide, *vis à vis* each patient, whether dying may be discussed openly or not. Since the patient's awareness of the situation fluctuates with his physical condition and his stage of adjustment to dying (Abrams, 1966), the team's decision should be reviewed and amended throughout the terminal period.

Where the team does not make a united decision to care for the patient in a consistent awareness context, ambiguous or contradictory communications to the patient are likely to complicate his terminal adjustment. In such a situation the patient has to bear the burden of protecting some of his caregivers and selecting others with whom he may discuss dying openly. Hence the need to assess and regulate aware-ness contexts is vital.

The social worker is in an ideal position to assist in these team de-cisions. Her skills in interviewing and in assessing personal capacities enable her to obtain information relevant to the decision. Her assess-ment of how the patient is likely to react to impending death is based, *inter alia,* on information concerning his reaction to former life crises and particularly to situations involving loss, or the death of a relative or friend.

(3) *Decoding the patient's behaviour*

The task of decoding the terminal patient's behaviour involves identi-fying in what stage of psychosocial adjustment to dying the patient is currently engaged and then alerting caregivers accordingly. It is valu-able, for example, to be able to assure the much-criticised doctor that the patient's discontent with his treatment may be an expression of his anger at the total situation, rather than a personal attack on that doctor. Once the doctor understands this interpretation, he is more likely to be able to tolerate such criticism and therefore no longer needs to avoid the patient, as he has previously been tempted to do.

In undertaking this task in terminal care work the social worker may at times be able to work with her counter-transference feelings (Salzberger-Wittenberg, 1970), that is, use her interaction with the team in relation to a particular patient in order to increase her understanding of the kind of feeling which the patient arouses in herself and others, and then to share her insight with her colleagues.

(4) *Ensuring the designation of a primary caregiver*
A patient who is preparing for separation and death is not in a position to have many new relationships thrust upon him. Where the caring team is extensive, it is unrealistic to expect each team member to interact with him at the level required to facilitate the resolution of his crisis. Consequently the team should elect one member to be designated 'primary caregiver' *vis à vis* each patient.

The presence of a primary caregiver does not absolve other team members of their responsibility for the patient's care. Colleagues continue their contacts, and the doctor in charge maintains overall responsibility for patient care. Meanwhile the primary caregiver undertakes the bulk of work to be done in the area of facilitating the patient's emotional, social and spiritual adjustment to death.

The task of ensuring that a primary caregiver is designated consists of proposing the procedure, assessing the most appropriate caregiver for the task, obtaining team agreement on the choice and communicating the outcome of the decision to all concerned. Basically this task involves facilitating the team's conscious acknowledgement of the need for a primary caregiver. The worker is often in a position to observe the patterns which emerge in assigning this task to team members. Where, for example, caregivers repeatedly absolve themselves of the task she may bring this action to their notice. After a primary caregiver has been designated she can ensure that the team undertakes to give that person the support needed to fulfil the role. In this regard, Morrissey (1963) writes that 'the [primary] therapist needs not only psychiatric consultation, but also the support and understanding of staff members who can help him make use of other sources of gratification.

The primary caregiver is not infrequently designated as such after 'selection' by the patient, who, as has already been stated, intuitively indicates with which team member he feels most comfortable in discussing his situation (Kübler-Ross, 1970a; Weisman, 1972a). Candidate team members for the role of primary caregiver may be, among others, a relative of the patient, the doctor, nurse, chaplain, psychologist, psychiatrist, social worker, or other paramedical staff.* In cases where the social worker is not the appropriate person for the task, her role will be to lend support to the team member so designated.

* See the following for references to these professionals in the role of primary caregiver to the terminal patient. Quint, 1965, 1967 and 1972; Carlozzi, 1968; Lasagna, 1969; Le Shan, 1969; Norton, 1969; Cavanagh, 1971; and Hertzberg, 1972.

(5) *Focusing on the feelings which colleagues experience in relation to their work*

Many writers have noted that doctors and nurses experience feelings of frustration, anger, threat, guilt, impotence, despair, failure and fear in relation to their work with the dying patient. Consequently, common staff reactions to terminal care work include indifferent or inept management, or avoidance of the situation (Feifel, 1963; Sudnow, 1967; Hinton, 1968a; Lasagna, 1969; and Cramond, 1970; among others). Another consequence, as Weisman (1972a and b) has observed, is that these uncomfortable feelings are often communicated to the patient.

In order to ensure optimal patient care therefore caregivers need to be aware of their feelings and support each other in dealing with them. The question of one team member's right to deal with the feelings of her co-workers has raised considerable controversy. Were it to be the social worker, some colleagues would criticise her for wielding too extensive a mandate. It is my contention however that the social worker, by virtue of her training, is one of several staff members who *is* equipped to initiate and facilitate this area of work.

Several writers support the case for the social worker's role in this interpretive activity. For example, Pincus and Minhan (1973) view focusing on the feelings which colleagues experience in relation to their work as one aspect of work with non-clients in the situation. It constitutes a task encompassed within the activity they term 'facilitating interaction within resource systems'. In similar vein McCollum and Schwarz (1972), writing of the related topic of grief work, describe the social worker's role as, *inter alia*, that of consultant to the caregiving team. Peretz (1972) also supports the social worker in this role. The psychosocial therapist in terminal care should work with primary, secondary and tertiary patients. She should render a direct clinical service to primary patients and in order to lessen the likelihood of maladaptation affecting others in the terminal care community she should also perform a preventive service with secondary and tertiary patients in the situation. It becomes clear, therefore, that the 'patient' approached by the social worker may at various times be the dying person, his family members, other patients, or the staff in the setting.

Interpretive or interdisciplinary work in terminal care may therefore routinely include the social worker's efforts to support her colleagues in dealing with their feelings concerning their work. It should however be stressed that colleagues should not become the social worker's clients; instead she should use her social work skills to promote a better understanding and acceptance of feelings as they affect the work at hand. At the same time it must be emphasised that this task is likely to be undertaken reciprocally by many members in the caregiving team. It is possible however that on account of the social worker's training she is one of several team members likely to be especially equipped to focus on the feelings aroused in colleagues by terminal care work.

The content of this task may include handling and supporting feelings aroused by terminal care work, organising other supportive resources for the team as a group and/or individually (for example, psychiatric consultation as described by Hertzberg 1972, or a 'psychological' autopsy as undertaken by Weisman and Kastenbaum (1968), and facilitating the team's optimal use of such resources.

Case illustration 25: an opportunity to focus interpretive work on the feelings of a colleague

In the midst of a busy outpatient chemotherapy clinic, after seeing a patient who had deteriorated noticeably in the past week, a consultant physician asked the social worker: 'Can you take it any longer? I can't. I'm ready to give up, after four years here . . . What's the use? All our patients die eventually.' As he spoke, he looked and sounded depressed. He had red eyes, which he rubbed. After a pause he continued: 'B— (another doctor) also feels it. He's changed too; I can see it . . .'

In response, the worker suggested that they needed to discuss these issues, and asked him when it would be convenient. He readily suggested a suitable time. They met a few days later, for forty-five minutes, during which time the worker helped the doctor to focus on his feelings concerning his work, to reaffirm the purpose and value of such work and to formulate criteria for assessing what terminal care work could achieve in the health care system. The worker also suggested that the doctor might benefit from regular discussions of that nature and recommended a clinical psychologist whom he might wish to use as a consultant for his work with terminal patients.

This brief illustration demonstrates how interpretive work between social work and the health disciplines may be initiated. Many opportunities to focus on the feelings of colleagues arise through spontaneous interaction between team members. The social worker should use such opportunities for this purpose. Alternatively, formal team meetings may also be used in this way. An informal opportunity for interpretive work, as reflected in this illustration, may be used to arrange regular consultation sessions for the team member in question, possibly with the social worker as consultant.

The episode discussed in the illustration relates to the question of the worker's right to work with the feelings of her colleagues. By responding spontaneously to an informal situation the social worker met the need of her colleague. She did not treat him as her client but reacted to a communication of feeling and referred him to another resource for more regular help regarding his work. Her role lay in helping her colleague to acknowledge his feelings in relation to his work (a task not dissimilar to that of the supervisor in social work).

(6)   *Guiding colleagues in the selection and referral of terminal patients*
       for social work intervention
Aiding colleagues to select and refer patients for social work service
poses difficulties for practitioners in many settings. It is easy to say
that the team needs to decide on its criteria. It is far more difficult to
say how this might be accomplished. Indeed, perhaps there are no
recipe-like answers at all. Certainly if they exist I am, at present, un-
aware of them. Hence my suggestion to fellow practitioners is to contain the anxieties involved and persevere towards their resolution while
at the same time using the struggle to remain in touch with what the
patient is probably enduring.

Many complicated issues are involved: patient need, scarce resources, quality of service, accountability, role clarity, priorities, referral procedures and team agreement or conflict in these areas. However, the social worker can appropriately place on the whole caring
team the onus of defining team roles and formulating a policy with
regard to eligibility for the various services. She would then need to
guide them in deciding upon their criteria for social work referrals.
For example, accountability demands that our help is focused on
amenable target groups – and scarce resources require us to accept that
it is not possible to offer social services to every terminal patient in the
community. But then – happily – nor does every patient need social
work aid in the resolution of the crisis.

How then does the social worker decide on the difficult question of
who would benefit from her aid? Three steps seem to be involved,
although their order is not fixed: the social worker needs to clear her
own thinking, to communicate her views to the team and to negotiate
until agreement is reached between them. In some cases it is only in
discussion with the team that her own ideas will be clarified. There is
no easy answer. However, the following criteria – applicable to many
helping professions – may be useful as a guide:

  (i)   those who seek aid, that is, those who can acknowledge a difficulty
        and take steps to obtain some help, are most likely to benefit
        from it;
 (ii)   those who are mentally healthy, or mature, may not need any
        outside intervention;
(iii)   those who are too disturbed by what life has had to offer may not
        benefit from social work help even if it is available to them.

It thus seems that several questions are involved: who should receive
the aid, how to ensure that he does receive it, and then, does he benefit
from it?
    The health care team needs to air these questions and take the views
of all the members into account. The social worker is one of several

participants whose task lies in ensuring that the questions are raised, discussed openly and that some decisions and policies result as a guideline to them all. For example, answers are needed with regard to when to withdraw, when to concentrate efforts mainly on the families, when not to get involved at all and/or whether to refer in terms of what help is available or only in terms of greatest patient need.

How then does the team assess which patients fall into each of the above three categories? Again, the social worker can help them to identify the factors involved. Some pertain to patient need and some to dynamics which the team members bring to the situation. Let us deal with patient need first. Factors which indicate mental health and mature functioning remain a guide. For example, a positive self image, some realistic problem-solving capacities, stable family relationships, a steady work record, a not too disrupted childhood, inner resources to cope with stress (for example, a positive philosophy of life, or religious faith) and outer supports, for example, family, friends, work, recreational outlets, food, shelter and clothing may all be strengths in the situation.

The absence of too many of these factors may indicate a patient too deprived, damaged or disturbed to respond to social work. In addition, patterns of coping with past life tasks, especially those involving loss, will indicate the patient's capacity to cope now and to use available help. In this sense the patient's ability to acknowledge his need, problem or difficulty becomes a crucial factor in deciding whether he will benefit from social work help or not, since the patient who does not acknowledge a problem is unlikely to work on it.

Thus the dying patient who is beset by too many problems and needs is unlikely to seek aid or benefit from it, while the patient who is immobilised on only one or two dying tasks may well benefit from social work intervention. In other words, the patient who has been disturbed and unmotivated in life is unlikely to change that pattern much in death, while the patient who has been relatively healthy in life is likely to grow even in dying, and *is* likely to work with the social worker to maximise this growth. Indeed such a patient may master his situation without social work – or any other human – aid. It is thus the middle group of not too disturbed, but not too healthy, patients which is likely to benefit most from social work aid and which colleagues should be encouraged to refer.

Criteria that are likely to prove useful in selecting patients who may benefit from *social group work aid* include: a common disease or some common experience of disease and a desire to talk about this experience. These two factors are likely to promote group cohesiveness, and so enhance the potential of the group's effectiveness, far more than similar socio-economic factors or the like.

So far we have considered referral and benefits to the patient in terms of his characteristics. But several factors which the team and caregivers bring to the situation also affect decisions regarding who receives the service, how the referral is made and how beneficial it is: for example, role definitions, each member's security in his/her professional role and the team members' discomfort in working with death and dying. One option open to the team in this situation is to refer patients according to what help is available, rather than according to their needs. For example, if the social worker works well with one kind of patient it may prove economic to refer those patients who could benefit from her particular style, rather than those in greatest need. Or the patient may be referred in terms of agreed-upon role expectations. But for that to happen role definitions need to be agreed upon in the team. The social worker's view of what her profession has to offer to this situation, what anyone can do for this patient and what contribution she herself can make needs to be matched with the team's views. Do they recognise her contribution, refer patients for what she feels is appropriate, or for some magical service that neither she nor anyone else can offer? Conversely, are the team's expectations realistic in the situation whereas her skills are not equal to the task? While these issues remain unclear, with regard to every team member's role, confusion is likely to reign and the patient will either not be referred at all, or several team members will duplicate their efforts to meet his needs.

One outcome of role confusion is that the social worker's conflicting needs to prove her own contribution to her colleagues, or to hold up a consistent picture for her profession's place in multidisciplinary practice, may influence her to encourage referrals which are not amenable to social work aid. Unless she feels comfortable in acknowledging that social work cannot 'put all things right', and is sure that social work aid is not appropriate to all patients, she will be tempted to accept 'impossible' referrals and to spend her scarce resources ineffectively.

Sometimes even after role negotiations referrals remain unclear because unconscious fears and attitudes to dying intervene. When this occurs patients are referred in order for the team to avoid the discomfort of working with dying patients. For example, in selecting terminal patients for social work help, the team members may refer not those patients who will benefit but those who are most threatening to them, hoping in this way to absolve themselves of responsibility for such patients. In response the social worker's interpretive task can lie in helping them to acknowledge the criteria they have used for the selection of that patient for additional psychosocial aid.

Thus, in summary, the patient may be referred because he needs help, requests help, is assessed to be likely to benefit from the service, because the service is available (rather than appropriate), because the social worker works well with that kind of patient, because the team thinks that the social worker solicits the referral and/or because no one else in the team wants to, or is able to deal with him. Whichever of these many factors are involved, the referral is likely to prove more effective if the reasons have been agreed upon by both the patient and the team members. Without formulated criteria, barriers of conflicting expectations, blurred role boundaries and unclear goals are likely to interfere both with the team's communication and the direct help eventually given to the patient.

COMMUNITY WORK

In addition to work within the health care system an effective service may need to be extended beyond the home or hospital. Community work in terminal care thus focuses on the patient in relation to the broader environment in which his dying takes place.

The link between clinical and community work comes not because death is a community problem to be solved, but by combining the private troubles of one individual terminal patient and his family in order to make public issues of their management in the community as a whole (Pincus and Minahan, 1973). Thus, as in other fields of social work, a balance needs to be maintained between the patient's needs and the resources available to meet them. Where services do not exist social work skill is needed in the imaginative and timely use of available scarce resources, in order to make the most of them (Younghusband, 1973).

The content of community work may include, *inter alia*, public and professional education, efforts to influence health and welfare structures, policies and delivery systems, the development of new services and facilities, social advocacy and collaborative work with colleagues in the community. In executing any of these activities the social worker needs to focus her efforts on enlisting not only the participation of the providers of services, but also of their consumers – the terminal patient, his relatives, recently bereaved families, volunteers and citizens of the community as a whole (Ross and Lappin, 1967). This statement is not however meant to imply that the social worker involved in the direct care of the patient is necessarily in the best position to undertake all these activities as well, although she may sometimes be. Nevertheless she may need at least to consider them.

Again, the tasks involved are identified by Pincus and Minahan (1973) to help the worker identify from where problems may stem if she is not working fruitfully in this area. They may or may not be carried out by the worker who is simultaneously engaged in clinical work. No special modification is required in order to apply these social work tasks to the terminal care setting. Nor have any additional community work tasks specific to terminal care been identified.

The first step in community work is to identify the community's needs and to assess the resources available to meet them. For example, Pincus and Minahan (1973) provide us with a useful framework for this task.

(a) *Resources which are needed but do not exist*

  (i) Is there a hospice or similar specific terminal care hospital, day care facility, community service and/or consultant service in the community?
 (ii) Have any statistics been gathered to show the need for such facilities?
(iii) Do any preventive services exist in the community? (For example, early detection units for cancer of the cervix or breast)?
 (iv) Do services exist to aid families in grief?
  (v) What facilities exist to train those who care for the terminal patients, his relatives and people in mourning?
 (vi) Who in the community takes formal responsibility for terminal care? Has any policy been formulated in this regard? Does the denial of death in contemporary Western society partly explain its absence?

(b) *Resources may exist, but not in sufficient numbers*

  (i) How many beds in the locality are allocated permanently for the care of terminal patients?
 (ii) To what extent have pain control techniques been developed by doctors in the community? Has such practice been inhibited on account of fears of inducing addiction?
(iii) To what extent have local medical practitioners explored and discussed the issue of telling the patient? Has any policy in this regard been formulated by any caregiving teams operating in the community?
 (iv) Where terminal care facilities exist in the community, are there sufficient for the whole population's need?

(c) *Resources may exist but be geographically, psychologically, or financially unsuitable to consumers*

  (i) Are terminal care facilities too costly for the average person to afford?
 (ii) Are services sited accessibly? If not, are transport facilities adequate?

(d) *Resources may exist but are not known about or present difficulty to the user*

  (i) Are terminal patients aware of the services available to them?

(e)   *Resources may exist, but their very operation creates new problems for the consumer*

(i)   How are the resources in the community co-ordinated? At the level of individual care are contradictory messages conveyed to the patient by different caregivers (thus complicating his dying work) because of poor co-ordination?

(ii) Is there continuity of care for the dying person, or in the course of his dying does he depend upon: general practitioners, radio-ologist, surgeon, personnel from different hospital departments and then perhaps general practitioners again? Does the lack of continuity of care complicate the patient's dying work, and make it difficult for caregivers to assess and monitor his adjustment to the situation, or plan appropriate intervention?

(iii) Do the role requirements of a terminal or a cancer patient present problems in a death-denying society? For example, do relatives avoid the services of the Marie Curie Foundation or National Society for Cancer Relief in an effort to protect the terminal patient from awareness of his terminal condition?

In response to identified areas of local need, priorities for action can be set. My own proposals are as follows.

Community work priority for terminal care
Generating awareness concerning terminal care may be decided on as one area of community work in which considerable effort is needed, among both lay and professional groups.

This decision may be taken because many health care professionals and non-professionals in the terminal care field can be involved in such an educational programme and can, hopefully, bring added understanding and skill to their work as a result. Creating public awareness can also motivate other people to participate in bringing about an effective terminal care service in that society. Community participation can thus be ensured and many different aspects of community work may result, for example, mobilising volunteers, fund-raising, pressing for more or better services and/or developing specific skills for terminal care, which can of course be used towards the care of other people as well.

Relevant target groups may include under- and postgraduates in health, education, welfare and theology, members of professional associations, workers in terminal care, grief work and related services, and interested citizens and community volunteers in churches, service societies, schools, parent–teacher associations and so on.

Such an education campaign may be offered under the joint auspices of the local university, hospital and/or similar educational authorities which carry considerable credibility and esteem in the community.

The process of a terminal care education campaign need not be presented in any detail, as I do not think that the execution of this social work function differs significantly from community work in any other field of social work. The teaching involved will be discussed as a separate social work function. The results of such a campaign are likely to be slow and not easily visible. So much more will probably need to be done. But at least the process will have been set in motion.

Indirect care on the patient's behalf may also necessitate some teaching – of colleagues, both professional and lay, and including the relatives of the dying person. The link between clinical work and teaching lies in the recognition that total patient care requires some knowledge and skills which various team members may not yet have developed. Again this social work function may or may not be undertaken by the same worker who is in direct contact with the patient. Other members of the team may do the teaching, while the social worker does the caring, or vice versa. Or it may be undertaken by several team members together. It is listed as a social work function to define the scope of a total terminal care service.

The aim of teaching is to equip caregivers to be of service to the person who is dying. Optimally, its goal is to return the care of the dying person to its former position in society – that of a natural life event to be managed at home, with concern and efficiency rather than with fuss and panic. Professional colleagues thus need to be taught to recognise a point at which cure is no longer a viable goal. Instead the task may need to be returned to the family and the community, while the team's role is one of accompanying the patient and/or supporting and guiding his lay caregivers.

Educating for terminal care involves both knowledge and skill: knowledge concerning the terminal crisis and skill in responding to the needs of the dying person. Hence this function needs to encompass both imparting knowledge and fostering the development of skill in others. As such it is likely to draw on principles from several bodies of knowledge, including adult education, learning theory, human growth and development, social work, communications theory and group dynamics. Educating for terminal care may be approached from several points of view: (a) as a compulsory, integral part of basic undergraduate training for relevant professionals (for example, nurses, doctors, chaplains, social workers and other paramedical staff), aimed at equipping them for work with people who may live or die; (b) as a specialised, postgraduate course, aimed at producing a new profession of terminal care experts who, by definition, absolve ordinary nurses, doctors and others of the task of caring for people who may not recover –

which view I have already disclaimed; or (c) as an adult education exercise, provided in response to a need, as a voluntary additional training opportunity for professional and lay caregivers.

My approach is to adopt the last alternative since in many countries in the world terminal care courses have not yet been established as an integral part of undergraduate training in medicine, nursing, social work or theology. In addition, training in response to the learner's identification of his own need avoids some of the resistance that is natural in this kind of learning. It also leaves him with responsibility for his own continued education, rather than encouraging dependence on the teacher, a delicate balance that requires the constant attention of the adult educator. Since teaching and learning skill in handling the dying person are internationally recognised assets in this field, it may be worthwhile outlining one educational opportunity which I have found effective.

A structure for a teaching–learning session: working with a dying person

Target group: This format may be used as an effective starting point for a wide variety of learners: professional or lay caregivers of any age, discipline, or experience, whether presently engaged in the task or in preparation for it. It may be offered under the auspices of an educational institution, hospital, church, community service, or similar body.

The trainer's objectives: By the end of this session participants will, to greater or lesser degrees, have

been exposed to some of the reactions and feelings experienced by a dying person and his family;
identified some of their preconceptions about a dying person;
distinguished between some of their stereotyped images and their reality experiences in relation to a dying person;
distinguished between imagining, seeing, thinking and feeling about a dying patient;
identified some of their own feelings about caring for a dying patient;
experienced some feelings around contravening a cultural norm by delving into a taboo topic;
identified and experienced some appropriate ways of responding to the feelings which may be expressed by a dying patient;
held in conscious awareness – however briefly – some of their feelings, fears and fantasies around their own death or dying;
tolerated a little closer contact with death and dying than before.

Since this educational event aims to teach some knowledge, attitudes and skills, the ideal structure for it is a group of six to ten people. It can also be managed in a class of up to forty learners, preferably sitting informally in a circle or circles. This learning may take the form of a single one-hour event, or if the objectives are to be fully met it may be extended into a course, the role-play sections being repeated, spread over several sessions, or over several whole days.

Programme Structure	Planning Comments
1 Hand out or display reference list and objectives [a].	a The learners can be freed from the anxiety of trying to master the theory in this hour.
2 *Introduction* State the purpose of the session and the form it is going to take, that is, that it will not be a lecture but a discussion in which learners may feel free to participate [b],	b Help the learners to tune in to the topic. Since many students are likely to come with expectations of being taught or of passive learning, the trainer may avoid later anxiety or confusion by sharing expectations at the outset. If both the content and the methods seem too unfamiliar to the learners, the trainer may negotiate both issues with the learners, and try to arrive at some areas of agreement. The absence of such a contract may inhibit learning.
introduce the 'trainer' [c] (myself) and	c Learners have a right to know the credentials and authority of the trainer. Credibility can enable trust and sufficient safety to risk learning. The manner in which the trainer introduces herself serves as a model for the learners and can set a standard for acceptance and the open expression of feeling and vulnerability in the session.
inquire if learners know who the other participants are. If not, they may introduce themselves to each other and to the trainer [d].	d Knowing who fellow learners are can also contribute to a climate necessary for learning.
3 Involve the learners in the subject, first via their senses, then their	

Programme Structure

intellect and then their emotions [e].

For example, brief participants: Picture, each one for yourself, preferably with closed eyes [f],

a dying patient... It may be someone known to you professionally or personally... [g]

someone who has died, or is dying, or it may be a picture that comes to your mind, not anyone in particular, but an image of 'a dying person'... [h]

What does he/she *look* like [i]?

What do you *think* he/she is experiencing, *feeling* or going through [j]?

Planning Comments

e If the teacher recognises that the topic may raise defences, it is worth approaching it gradually once some security and trust exists.

f Some learners may resist closing their eyes. Those who manage it often have a more vivid picture, and hence a fuller experience. The trainer may comment on the difficulty if no one does it.

g The trainer needs to move at the pace of the learners, to anticipate threat and approach gradually. At the same time, for those people who are ready for personal learning, the opportunity is given.

h Again the teacher can allow for learning at different levels and by so doing can make the point that there is not only one right answer, or right way to do the exercise or to learn. The analogy that accompanies this message is that there are many right ways of caring for a dying person.

i With the objectives of the session in mind, the trainer can structure and enable the learning.

j Awareness of the difference between what the learner *sees* and *thinks* the patient is enduring, and what the patient *is* actually feeling become apparent.

Programme Structure
What is he/she saying [k]?

What is being said to you [l]?

And what are you beginning to *feel* as you are there in the picture [m]?

4 Allow a silence for two to three minutes [n].

5 The trainer can then ask if anyone is ready to share his/her experience [o].

6 Some points to consider may include, for example, identifying how fear looks, how it is experienced, how it may be expressed – or disguised, how it makes *us* feel, what there is to be feared in dying and how we can respond, helpfully, to such situations [p].

Planning Comments
k There is room for projection or for reliving past experience(s).

l Gradually the learner's self can be brought into the experience.

m Lastly, the learner's feelings are touched on.

n Learners need time to absorb and experience the scene, and to stay with the feelings for a space.

o The discussion may be guided to cover each question, to highlight the differences between assumption and reality; looks, thoughts, feelings of others and our own; and to identify and balance the negatives and the positives in the situation. The group's dynamics can be observed and used to enable support, identification, sharing, learning and self-help.

p The acceptability of many points of view and of different responses is demonstrated.

One outcome of this exercise is the development of the terminal care skill of tolerating close contact with death and dying. My experience has been that this capacity is based largely upon the conviction that both positive and negative elements exist in the terminal situation. As long as learners are aware only of the negatives, working with dying people is likely to be uncomfortable and, often, avoided. Certainty that the balance exists, that growth *is* possible and has been observed and experienced by others in these circumstances, makes the whole situation more bearable. I think that it is vital to enable this point to emerge, preferably from the learners themselves.

Other *content* that usually needs to be covered includes the naturalness of death, preparation for dying as a life-task, the nature of the terminal crisis, the spiritual issues involved and how to respond to these issues, especially 'telling' the patient.

---

7 If there is time, a role-play can be used as an effective means of exploring the ideas kindled through the discussion.

8 *Evaluation and termination* [n]
The trainer may ask what has been learnt so far. Or, about ten minutes before the end, if a great deal of content has yet to be covered, she may give the learners a choice as to how best to use the little time they still have, and comment on the feelings involved in this process of deciding.

She may end on time, allow extra time, or give an experience of a sudden, unexpected ending.

If this is not a single learning event, facilitating some planning for future learning is appropriate.

n The trainer needs to be aware of the significance of modelling an ending.

This teaching format has proved useful, partly as it requires no audio-visual equipment or other teaching aids and hence can be presented in many different settings, without inconvenience or extra costs. Needless to say, it is most effective with groups who have themselves identified their need to know about terminal caring and have requested the learning.

Where the trainer is invited to come as an expert to provide answers to a passive audience which does not anticipate having to acknowledge the uncertainties and complexities in the situation, this format is unlikely to prove useful. Where such a clash of expectations occurs, the trainer may be tempted into the 'expert', lecturing role, as I have been on occasions, but my assessment is that little meaningful learning has occurred.

In summary, indirect or facilitative work in terminal care includes three social work functions which focus on the terminal patient in his relationship with significant persons and systems in his environment. Interpretive work between social work and the health professionals focuses on the patient in his relationship with the treatment team; community work focuses on his relationship with the broader community; and teaching aims to transmit terminal care knowledge and skill to all his caregivers. These three social work functions are considered to be vital to terminal care work in order to ensure total patient care.

CONCLUSION: THE RELEVANCE OF TERMINAL CARE
SERVICES TO OTHER SETTINGS

What can be said by way of modelling, since the reader has been alerted throughout the text to the fact that the feelings aroused by beginnings, middles and endings should be used to link the here and now with the process under discussion, dying? We have seen that the work involved in terminating all change efforts includes evaluation, disengaging from relationships and stabilising the change effort (Pincus and Minahan, 1973). We have recognised all these elements in the dying person's work, in his relatives' adjustment and in his caregivers' efforts.

Looking back on the task we find the preceding chapters reveal the ease of beginnings, the boredom of middles and the pain of endings. Happily the completion of this book echoes its message: the struggle is worth it and *does* lead on to new beginnings. Looking forward, stabilising the change effort demands that some attention is paid to ensuring that the achievements that have been made will endure. So in order to strengthen the life of this book it seems worthwhile to consider its relevance to situations other than the original one on which it has been based, that is, terminal care involving a malignant disease. For example, the service described could, with some modifications, apply also to:

1 terminal patients of all ages, including young children, suffering diseases other than malignant ones. There does also seem to be some application to events involving sudden, traumatic or unexpected deaths, even when there is little time for conscious preparation for dying. This approach can however certainly apply to the handling of relatives and friends who survive an unexpected death;
2 patients about to undergo major surgery, for whom preparation for dying may be unnecessary but may sometimes prove realistic and appropriate;
3 any other life-crisis which entails some adjustment or preparation work – as all life-tasks do require. The relevance here lies in acknowledging that the work involved in mastering any life-crisis has many common elements. I have found Kübler-Ross's paradigm of reactions a particularly helpful guide to many other situations of

change, growth, loss, or adaptation, and would offer her ideas to
caregivers in all sorts of circumstances;

4 bereavement or grief situations, one life-task for which there is
particular relevance in this approach. Since relatives and survivors
are making their adjustment to the event of death in many ways
similar to the work the patient has just completed, our ways of
responding to their plight are unlikely to differ from those outlined
for the dying person himself;

5 aged and aging people. All over the world the numbers of aged
people are increasing as medical technology enables greater
longevity. Many of them prepare for death over some years rather
than months as envisaged here. Nevertheless the process is the
same. Services to retired and pre-retirement groups are also likely
to find some relevance in what has been described for dying
persons;

6 situations involving endings of any kinds: relationships, cycles,
groups, organisations, projects, and so on. The work of protesting
against the necessity to part or end at all, evaluating what has
been achieved, grieving the anticipated separation, withdrawing
from the situation and stabilising what has been achieved, remains
the work of endings – irrespective of what it is that is reaching
completion (Smalley, 1970);

7 any health, welfare, or spiritual setting. If, as has been mentioned,
terminal care is viewed not as a new speciality, but as an integral
part of many caring professions, then this book has relevance for
all doctors, nurses, chaplains and paramedical professionals. It
will, hopefully, enhance their general caring for all their patients,
clients, or congregants;

8 situations of contemplated suicide. Once we understand that a fear
of death usually reflects a fear of some aspect of life, and that
suicidal intentions are often attempts to come to terms with death
fears, we can use our understanding of the terminal crisis in prevention and the treatment of suicidal patients;

9 decision-making regarding euthanasia. The difficulty involved in
such decisions lies in the complexity of these situations. But if we
can use our terminal care knowledge (to understand the perspectives of the various participants in the situation) and our terminal
care skill (to respond, in open communication to these many and
varied perspectives, bearing the total person in mind), it may be
possible to formulate some criteria for decisions in various circumstances, rather than working with intuition and uncertainty, as is
often the case at present;

10 a 'psychological autopsy' (Weisman and Kastenbaum, 1968) or a
'death investigation team'. Here, in addition to, or instead of, a
direct clinical service to the dying person, the team benefits from

a review, in perspective, of the deceased person's life situation. The caregivers try to discover a reliable relationship between preceding events and the terminal illness, and between the disease and the person who succumbed to it. The purposes of such multidisciplinary investigations are similar to those supporting all our interpretive work; they improve our understanding of the patient as a whole; they can minimise our discomfort after a death and our consequent blame of technical error, therapeutic deficiency and/or culpable ignorance. They also offer support to the whole team without challenging the doctor as the leader.

This book has been written as a spur to counteract the present neglect of the dying person. Rayner (1971) supports this demand to care for the patient who is approaching death when he writes that:

Those who break through this barrier of silence and talk to dying people rarely regret it. They feel they have contributed something to a person in his last days that is very intimate, and have been enriched themselves by the unforgettable, humbling experience of being with a person who has forsaken defences and illusions.

At the same time the caregiver's reward comes through increased awareness, at the very edge of life, that although death may have a sting, the grave does not have the victory.

The final plea for terminal care must, however, come on behalf of the dying person himself. In this regard, Milton (1973) writes: 'Kindly understanding by a team . . . will not eliminate the suffering of a patient, but will diminish it, – a modest achievement, but one worth obtaining.'

APPENDIX: LIST OF CASE ILLUSTRATIONS APPEARING IN THE TEXT

This list is presented to enable the reader to obtain an overall picture of some patients' adjustment to dying.

Patient	Case illustration	Page	Other page references to patient
Mrs E	(1) a terminal patient demonstrates acceptance of impending death	20	—
Mrs F	(2) inconsistent awareness of dying	24	—
Mrs I	(3) fluctuating hope	25	31, 91–4
Mr G	(4) a patient chooses to relinquish life	28	—
Mrs D	(5) a terminal patient relinquishes the will to live	29	59–65, 73, 74
Mr H	(6) death work incomplete: an inability to relinquish control	30	83
Mrs I	(7) a patient disengages herself from family responsibilities	31	25–7, 91–4
Mrs J	(8) separating the self from life	31	—
Mr K	(9) a patient's life culminates with achievement in dying	33	—
Mr N	(10) the social worker's ability to tolerate close contact with dying and death	51	—
Mrs D	(11) terminal crisis work in an initial interview with a patient	59	29, 73, 74
Mr A	(12) a patient's use of denial and the social worker's response	67	—
Mr B	(13) an isolated patient and the social worker's response	70	—
Mrs C	(14) an angry patient and the social worker's response	71	—
Mrs D	(15) a terminal patient bargains for more time	73	29, 59–65, 74
Mrs D	(16) a period of terminal de-		

Patient	Case illustration	Page	Other page references to patient
	pression and the social worker's response	74	29, 59–65, 73
Mrs O	(17) a patient who made no progress in her terminal crisis work despite social work intervention	76	—
Mr L	(18) terminal crisis work focusing on communication concerning the patient's awareness of impending death	78	88–9
Mr H	(19) the social worker attempts to facilitate the reversal and relinquishing processes involved in terminal adjustment	83	30
Mrs M	(20) the social worker aids the patient's detachment from relationships	85	—
Mr L	(21) terminal crisis work focusing on spiritual issues	88	78–82
Mrs I	(22) adjustment to the terminal situation, motivated by faith	91	25–7, 31
Mr D	(23) terminal crisis work with a relative of a patient	97	—
	(24) interpretive work between the social worker and a health professional (ward sister)	108	—
	(25) an opportunity to focus interpretive work on the feelings of a colleague	114	—

SELECT BIBLIOGRAPHY

Abrams, R. D. (1951), 'Social casework with cancer patients', *Social Casework*, vol. 10, pp. 425–32.

Abrams, R. D. (1966), 'The patient with cancer – his changing pattern of communication', *New England Journal of Medicine*, vol 274, pp. 317–22.

Abrams, R. D. (1971), 'Denial and depression in the terminal care patient – a clue for management', *Psychiatric Quarterly*, vol. 45, no. 3, pp. 394–404.

Abrams, R. D. (1972), 'The responsibility of social work in terminal cancer', in Schoenberg *et al.* (1972), pp. 173–84.

Abrams, R. D. (1974), *Not Alone with Cancer* (Springfield, Illinois: Charles C. Thomas).

Anthony, S. (1972), *The Discovery of Death in Childhood and After* (New York: Basic Books).

Autton, M. (1969), *The Pastoral Care of the Dying* (London: SPCK).

Bailey, M. (1959), 'A survey of the social needs of patients with incurable lung cancer', *The Almoner*, vol. 11, pp. 379–91.

Balint, M. (1968), *The Doctor, His Patient and the Illness* (London: Pitman).

Barrett, S. W. (1962), *Deathbed Visions* (London: Methuen).

Benton, R. G. (1978), *Death and Dying: Principles and Practices in Patient Care* (New York: Van Nostrand Reinhold).

Bermann, E. (1973), *Scapegoat. The Impact of Death Fear on an American Family* (Ann Arbor, Michigan: University of Michigan Press).

Birley, M. F. 1960), 'Terminal care', *The Almoner*, vol. 13, pp. 86–97.

Brim, O. G., Freeman, H. E., Levine, S., and Scotch, N. A. (eds) (1970), *The Dying Patient* (New York: Russell Sage Foundation).

Burton, L. (ed.) (1974), *Care of the Child Facing Death* (London: Routledge & Kegan Paul).

Butrym, Z. (1967), *Social Work in Medical Care* (London: Routledge & Kegan Paul).

Byrne, P. S., and Long, B. E. L. (1973), *Learning to Care: Person to Person* (London: Churchill, Livingstone & Edenborough).

Caplan, G. (1964), *Principles of Preventive Psychiatry* (London: Tavistock).

Caplan, G. (1970), *Theory and Practice of Mental Health Consultation* (London: Tavistock).

Cappon, D. (1961), 'The psychology of dying', *Pastoral Psychology* (February); repr. in Ruitenbeek (1969), pp. 61–72.

Carlozzi, C. G. (1968), *Death and Contemporary Man: The Crises of Terminal Illness* (Grand Rapids, Michigan: William B. Eerdmans).

Cartwright, A., Hockey, L., and Anderson, J. L. (1973), *Life Before Death* (London: Routledge & Kegan Paul).

Cavanagh, J. R. (1971), 'The chaplain and the dying patient', *Hospital Progress,* vol. 52 (November), pp. 35–40.

Chambers, M. (1974), 'Aspects of social work on a cancer research and treatment unit in a London teaching hospital', *British Journal of Social Work*, vol. 4, no. 2 (Summer), pp. 413–62.

Cockerill, E. (1937), 'The social worker looks at cancer', *The Family* vol. 17, pp. 326–9.

Collipp, P. J. (1969), 'The efficacy of prayer: a triple-blind study', *Medical Times*, vol. 97 (May), pp. 201–4.

Conan Doyle, Sir A. (1926), *History of Spiritualism* (London: Cassell).

Cooper, H. (1973), 'The psychological needs and care of the dying patient', *South African Medical Journal*, vol. 47 (September), pp. 1711–14.

Cramond, W. A. (1970), 'Psychotherapy of the dying patient', *British Medical Journal*, vol. 3 (August), pp. 389–93.

Cronk, H. M. (1972), 'This business of dying', *Nursing Times*, vol. 68 (August 31), p. 1100.

Daniel, M. P. (1973), 'The social worker's role in the care of the dying', *British Medical Journal*, no. 1 (6 January), pp. 36–8.

Department of Health and Social Security (1973), *Care of the Dying*, Reports on Health and Social Subjects, no. 5 (London: HMSO).

Dewi-Rees, W. (1972), 'The distress of dying', *British Medical Journal*, vol. 3, pp. 105–7.

Dominian, J. (1970), 'Facing death', in Shotter, E. F. (ed.), *Matters of Life and Death* (London: Darton, Longman & Todd), pp. 24–7.

Erikson, E. H. (1950), *Childhood and Society* (Harmondsworth: Penguin).

Falkson, G., et al. (1973), 'Report on carcinoma chemotherapy research carried out during 1972', *South African Cancer Bulletin*, vol. 17, no. 4 (December), pp. 125–77.

Farberow, N. L. (ed. (1963), *Taboo Topics* (New York: Atherton Press).

Feifel, H. (1963), 'Death', in Farberow (1963).

Feifel, H. (ed.) (1965), *The Meaning of Death* (New York: McGraw-Hill).

Fischel, E. (1937), 'What the social worker can do about cancer', *The Family*, vol. 17, pp. 322–6.

Foster, Z. P. L. (1965), 'How social work can influence hospital management of fatal illness', *Social Work* (New York), vol. 10, no. 4 (October), pp. 30–5.

Fox, E. G., Nelson, M. A., and Bolman, W. M. (1969), 'The termination process: a neglected dimension in social work', *Social Work* (New York), vol. 14, no. 4 (October), pp. 53–63.

Fulton, R. (ed.) (1966), *Death and Identity* (New York: Wiley).

Fulton, R., and Fulton, J. (1971), 'A psychosocial aspect of terminal care: anticipatory grief', *Omega*, vol. 2, no. 2 (May), pp. 99–100.

Garrad, J. (1968), 'The right to die', *Medical Social Work*, vol. 20, no. 10 (March), pp. 327–30.

Glaser, B. G., and Strauss, A. L. (1966), *Awareness of Dying* (London: Weidenfeld & Nicolson).

Goldberg, S. T. (1973), 'Family tasks and reactions in the crisis of death', *Social Casework*, vol. 54, no. 7, pp. 398–405.

Goldstein, E. G. (1973), 'Social casework with the dying person', *Social Casework*, vol. 54, no. 10, pp. 601–9.

Gorer, G. (1965), *Death, Grief and Mourning in Contemporary Britain* (London: Cresset Press).

134   TOWARDS DEATH WITH DIGNITY

Green, B. R., and Irish, D. P. (1971), *Death Education – Preparation for Living* (Cambridge: Schenkman).
Group for the Advancement of Psychiatry (1965), *Death and Dying: Attitudes of Patient and Doctor*, Vol. 5, Symposium No. 11 (New York: GAP).
Group for the Advancement of Psychiatry (1973), *The Right to Die: Decisions and Decision Makers*, Vol. 8 (New York: GAP).
Hamovitch, M. B. (1963), 'Research interviewing in terminal illness', *Social Work* (New York), vol. 8, no. 1 (April), pp. 4–9.
Hegy, R. (1964), *A Witness Through the Centuries* (London: Psychic Press).
Henke, E. (1972), 'The purpose of life', *Omega*, vol. 3, no. 2 (May), p. 163.
Hertzberg, L. J. (1972), 'Cancer and the dying patient', *American Journal of Psychiatry*, vol. 128, no. 7 (January), pp. 806–10.
Herzog, E. (1966), *Psyche and Death* (London: Hodder & Stoughton).
Heusinkveld, K. B. (1972), 'Cues to communication with the terminal cancer patient', *Nursing Forum*, vol. 11, no. 11, pp. 105–13.
Hineman, J. H. (1971), 'Counselling with the terminally ill: a clinical study', PhD thesis (Educational Psychology), University of Utah, USA.
Hinton, J. (1968a), *Dying* (Harmondsworth: Penguin).
Hinton, J. (1968b), 'The dying and the doctor' in Toynbee (1968), ch. 10.
Hinton, J. (1973), 'Bearing cancer', *British Journal of Medical Psychology*, vol. 46, pp. 105–13.
Hutchnecker, A. A. (1959), 'Personality factors in dying patients', in Feifel (1959), pp. 237–50.
Jablon, R., and Volk, H. (1960), 'Revealing diagnosis and prognosis to cancer patients', *Social Work* (New York), vol. 5, no. 2, pp. 51–7.
Jenkins, D. H. (undated), *How to Teach Adults* (Washington, DC: Adult Education Association of USA).
Kalish, R. A. (1969), 'The effects of death upon the family', in L. Pearson (1969), pp. 79–107.
Kalish, R. A. (1970), 'The onset of the dying process', *Omega*, vol. 1, no. 1 (February), pp. 57–69.
Kalish, R. A. (1972), 'Of social values and the dying: a defence of disengagement', *Family Co-ordinator*, vol. 21, no. 1 (January), pp. 81–94.
Kastenhaum, R. (1966), 'Death and responsibility', *Psychiatric Opinion*, no. 3 (August), pp. 28–34.
Kastenbaum, R., and Aisenberg, R. (1972), *The Psychology of Death* (New York: Springer).
Kelly, W. D., and Freisen, S. R. (1950), 'Do cancer patients want to be told?', *Surgery*, vol. 27, no. 6, pp. 822–6.
Kennedy, N. E. (1960), *Helping the Dying Patient and His Family, Part III* (New York: National Association of Social Workers), pp. 23–31.
Killick, F. (1968), 'Casework with patients living with cancer', *Medical Social Work*, vol. 21, no. 1 (April), p. 16.
Knapp, V. S., and Hansen, H. (1973), 'Helping the parents of children with leukaemia', *Social Work* (New York), vol. 18, no. 4 (July), pp. 70–5.
Kübler-Ross, E. (1970a), *On Death and Dying* (London: Tavistock).
Kübler-Ross, E. (1970b), 'Psychotherapy for the dying patient', *Current Psychiatric Therapies*, vol. 10, pp. 110–17.

Kübler-Ross, E. (1971), 'What is it like to be dying?', *American Journal of Nursing*, vol. 71, no. 1 (January), pp. 54–60.

Kübler-Ross, E. (1972), 'Hope and the dying patient', in Schoenberg *et al.* (1972), pp. 221–5.

Kübler-Ross, E. (1974), *Questions and Answers on Death and Dying* (London: Collier Macmillan).

Lack, S., and Lamerton, R. (eds) (1974), *The Hour of Our Death* (London: Chapman).

Lang, P. A., and Oppenheimer, J. R. (1968), 'The influence of social work when parents are faced with the fatal illness of a child', *Social Casework*, vol. 49, no. 3 (March), pp. 161–6.

Lasagna, L. (1969), 'The doctor and the dying patient', *Journal of Chronic Diseases*, vol. 22 (July), pp. 68–9.

Le Shan, L. (1969), 'Psychotherapy and the dying patient', in L. Pearson (1969), pp. 28–9.

Le Shan, L., and Le Shan, E. (1969), 'Psychotherapy with the patient with a limited life span', in Ruitenbeek (1969), pp. 106–15.

Leech, The (1977), 'The dying patient', *Journal of the University of Witwatersrand Medical School*, vol. 47, no. 3.

Leslie, R. C. (1960), *Helping the Dying Patient and His Family, Part I* (New York: National Association of Social Workers), pp. 11–15.

Lindemann, E. (1944), 'Symptomatology and management of acute grief', *American Journal of Psychiatry*, vol. 101, pp. 141–9.

Lodge, Sir Oliver (1952), *Ether and Reality* (London: Hodder & Stoughton).

MacLaurin, H. (1959), 'In the hour of their going forth', *Social Casework*, vol. 40, no. 3, pp. 136–41.

Marcovitz, E. (1973), 'What is the meaning of death to the dying person and his survivors?', *Omega*, vol. 4, no. 1, pp. 13–25.

McCollum, A. T., and Schwartz, A. H. (1972), 'Social work and the mourning parent', *Social Work* (New York), vol. 17, no. 1, pp. 25–36.

Menzies, Isabel E. P. (1970), *A Case-Study in the Functioning of Social Systems as a Defence against Anxiety* (London: Tavistock).

Milton, G. W. (1973), 'Contemporary themes: thoughts in mind of a person with cancer', *British Medical Journal*, no. 4 (October), pp. 221–3.

Moody, R. A. (1976), *Life after Life* (New York: Bantam Books).

Morrissey, J. R. (1963), 'A note on interviews with children facing imminent death', *Social Casework*, vol. 44 (June), pp. 343–5.

Muller, A. (1967), 'Terminale Sorg', in Theron and Muller (1967), pp. 60–5.

National Association of Social Workers (1960), *Helping the Dying Patient and His Family* (New York: NASW).

Norton, J. (1969), 'Treatment of a dying patient', in Ruitenbeek (1969), pp. 19–38.

Nursing Outlook (1972), 'Notes of a dying professor', *Nursing Outlook*, vol. 20, no. 8 (August), pp. 502–6.

Olin, H. S. (1972), 'A proposed model to teach medical students the care of the dying patient', *Journal of Medical Education*, vol. 47 (July), pp. 564–7.

Olsen, R. (1973), 'From the medical journals', *Social Work Today*, vol. 3, no. 24, pp. 17–18.

Oppenheimer, J. R. (1967), 'Use of crisis intervention in casework with the cancer patient and his family', *Social Work* (New York), vol. 12, no. 2 April), pp. 44–52.

Osis, K. (1961), *Deathbed Observations by Physicians and Nurses* (New York: Parapsychology Foundation).

Oler, Sir William (1906), *Science and Immortality* (Boston, Mass.: Houghton Mifflin).

Parkes, C. Murray (1972), *Bereavement: Studies of Grief in Adult Life* (London: Tavistock).

Pearson, L. (ed.), *Death and Dying* (Cleveland, Ohio: Case Western Reserve University Press).

Pearson, N. (1954), 'Casework in terminal illness in Great Britain', *The Almoner*, vol. 6, no. 11, pp. 448–91.

Peretz, D. (1972), 'Psychotherapy workshop', in Schoenberg *et al.* (1972), pp. 370–3.

Pettes, D. (1967), *Supervision in Social Work* (London: Allen & Unwin).

Pilsecker, C. (1975), 'Help for the dying', *Social Work* (New York), vol 20, no. 3, pp. 190–4.

Pincus, A., and Minahan, A. (1973), *Social Work Practice: Model and Method* (Itasca, Illinois: Peacock).

Player, A. (1954), 'Casework in terminal illness', *The Almoner*, vol. 6, no. 11 (February), pp. 447–88.

Poss, S. (1975), 'Patients in terminal care: a social work response', MA dissertation (Social Work), University of the Witwatersrand, Johannesburg.

Poss, S. (1980), 'How the terminal patient accepts dying', *Patient Counselling and Health Education*, vol. 2, no. 2, pp. 72–7.

Prentiss, E. (undated), *Stepping Heavenward* (London: Ward, Lock & Tyler).

Quint, J. C. (1965), 'Institutionalized practices of informational control', *Psychiatry*, vol. 28 (May, pp. 119–33.

Quint, J. C. (1967), *The Nurse and the Dying Patient* (New York: Macmillan).

Quint Benoliel, J. (1972), 'Nursing care for the terminal patient: a psychosocial approach', in Schoenberg *et al.* (1972), pp. 145–61.

Rapoport, L. (ed.) (1963a), *Consultation in Social Work Practice* (New York: National Association of Social Workers).

Rapoport, L. (1963b), 'Consultation: an overview', in Rapoport (1963a), pp. 7–20.

Rapoport, L. (1965), 'The state of crisis: some theoretical considerations', in Parad, H. J. (ed.) (1965), *Crisis Intervention: Selected Readings* (New York: Family Services Association of America), pp. 22–31.

Rapoport, L. (1970), 'Crisis intervention as a mode of brief treatment', in Roberts and Nee (1970), pp. 265–312.

Rayner, E. (1971), *Human Development* (London: Allen & Unwin).

Roberts, R. W., and Nee, R. H. (eds) (1970), *Theories of Social Casework* (Chicago: University of Chicago Press).

Rosenthal, H. R. (1957), 'Psychotherapy for the dying', *American Journal of Psychotherapy* (July); repr. in Ruitenbeek (1969).

Rosenthal, H. R. (1963), 'The fear of death as an indispensable factor in psychotherapy', *American Journal of Psychotherapy* (October); repr. in Ruitenbeek (1969), pp. 116–82.

Ross, M. G., and Lappin, B. W. (1967), *Community Organization: Theory, Principles and Practice* (New York: Harper & Row).

Ruitenbeek, H. M. (ed.) (1969), *Death: Interpretations* (New York: Delta Books).

Salzberger-Wittenberg, I. (1970), *Psycho-Analytic Insight and Relationships: A Kleinian Approach* (London: Routledge & Kegan Paul).

Saunders, C. (1965), 'The last stages of life', *American Journal of Nursing*, vol. 65 (March), pp. 70–5.

Saunders, C. (1966a), 'Death and responsibility: a medical director's view of death', *Psychiatric Opinion*, no. 3 (August), pp. 28–34.

Saunders, C. (1966b), 'The concerns of the patient', *Contact* (18 October), p. 13.

Saunders, C. (1972), 'A therapeutic community: St Christopher's Hospice', in Schoenberg *et al.* (1972), pp. 275–89.

Saunders, C. (1976), *Care of the Dying*, repr. from *Nursing Times* (London: Macmillan Journals).

Schoenberg, B. and Carr, A. (1972), 'Educating the health professional in the psychosocial care of the terminally ill', in Schoenberg *et al.* (1972), pp. 3–18.

Schoenberg, B., Carr, A. C., Peretz, D., and Kutscher, A. H. (eds) (1970), *Loss and Grief: Psychosocial Management in Medical Practice* (New York: Columbia University Press).

Schoenberg, B., Carr, A. C., Peretz, D., and Kutscher, A. H. (eds) (1972), *Psychosocial Aspects of Terminal Care* (New York: Columbia University Press).

Smalley, R. E. (1970), 'The functional approach to casework practice', in Roberts and Nee (1970), pp. 77–128.

Snelling, J. (1966), 'Grief reactions in the field of medical social work', *Case Conference*, vol. 2, pp. 2–8.

Spoor, J. M. (1975), 'Terminal illness: some facts and feelings', *Social Work Today*, vol. 5, no. 23 (20 February), pp. 702–7.

Stewart, J. (1970), 'Counselling as an experience of dependence', MA dissertation (Social Work), University of the Witwatersrand, Johannesburg.

Sudnow, D. (1967), *Passing On: The Social Organization of Dying* (Englewood Cliffs, NJ: Prentice-Hall).

Theron, E., and Muller, A. (eds) (1967), *Maatskaplike Aspekte van Siekte en Gesondheid* (Stellenbosch: Universiteits-Uitgewers en Boekhandel).

Tileston, M. W. (ed.) (1948), *Daily Strengths for Daily Needs* (London: Methuen).

Tilley, M. (1962), 'Religion and the social worker', *Social Work* (United Kingdom), vol. 19, no. 2 (April), pp. 7–10.

Tillich, P. (1959), 'The eternal now', in Feifel (1959), pp. 30–8.

Towle, C. (1945), *Common Human Needs* (New York: National Association of Social Workers).

Toynbee, A. (ed.) (1968), *Man's Concern with Death* (London: Hodder & Stoughton).

Vernick, J., and Karon, MM. (1965), 'Who's afraid of death on a leukemia ward?', *American Journal of Diseases of Children*, vol. 109, pp. 393–7.

Vernon, G. (1970), *Sociology of Death: An Analysis of Death-Related Behaviour* (New York: Ronald Press).

Wahl, C. W. (1966), 'The fear of death', in Fulton (1966), pp. 56–66.

Weisberg, L. M. (1974), 'Casework with the terminally ill', *Social Casework,* vol. 55, no. 6, pp. 337–42.

Weisman, A. D. (1972a), *On Dying and Denying: A Psychiatric Study of Terminality* (New York: Behavioural Publications).

Weisman, A. D. (1972b), 'Psychosocial considerations in terminal care', in Schoenberg *et al.* (1972), pp. 162–72.

Weisman, A. D., and Kastenbaum, R. (1968), *The Psychological Autopsy – A Study of the Terminal Phase of Life,* Community Mental Health Journal Monograph No. 4 (New York: Behavioural Publications).

Young, P. (1967), *The Student and Supervision in Social Work Education* (London: Routledge & Kegan Paul).

Younghusband, E. (1973), 'The future of social work', *Social Work Today,* vol. 4, no. 2 (April), pp. 33–6.

PUBLICATION DEALING SPECIFICALLY WITH ISSUES IN DYING, DEATH AND TERMINAL CARE

Omega, Baywood Publishing Co. Inc., 120 Marine St, Farmingdale, New York, NY 11735, USA. Editor: Dr R. J. Kastenbaum.

INDEX

manipulation of, by patient, *case illus. of* 70–1
primary caregiver within, designation of 4
and social work referrals, criteria for 115–18
social worker support for 107–18
and spiritual issues, discussion of 87
training for 121–7
caring professions/professionals:
anger against 15, 37; *case illus. of* 55, 72
difficulties of 5, 43, 44
in-service training for 43–4
as primary caregivers 14
relevance of terminal care services to 128
and religious issues 87–8
and terminal care, context of within xii
withdrawal from patient by, *case illus. of* 70
see also social work; social worker
caring skills 43–57; *case illus. of* 51–6
Carlozzi, C. G. 3, 25, 32, 33, 39n, 43, 89, 112n
Cavanagh, J. R. 112n
Chambers, M. 105
children 40, 107, 127
Cockerill, E. 105
collusion, *see* game playing
community work xiii, 9–10, 11, 107, 118–21, 127
and available resources 118
assessment of, framework for 119–20
caregiving team in 4–5
content of 118
priority action in, proposals for 120
public participation in 120
tasks of 118
consultation/supervision 9, 11
control:
of feelings, *case illus. of* 67–9, 91–4
over life 16, 26, 51, 61; *case illus. of* 76, 83, 91
relinquishment of 27, 29–30; *case illus. of* 29, 52, 83–5, 91
inability to achieve, *case illus. of* 30
over terminal crisis 99; *case illus. of* 83
counselling *see* social work interven-

tion; social worker; terminal care work
Cramond, W. A. 13, 77, 110, 113

Daniel, M. P. 39n, 95, 104
death work *see* dying work
decathexis 19, 30
deception 13, 14, 22, 23, 37, 48, 95, 96
denial of death:
by caregivers 22, 45, 66, 77, 109
by patient 12–13, 14, 26, 34, 35, 60; *case illus. of* 51–6 *passim*, 67–9, 76, 78–9, 81, 83, 88–90 *passim*
social worker's response to 10, 65–9; *case illus. of* 67–9, 83–4
verbal expression of 13
by relatives 37
depression:
preparatory:
of caregivers 114
of patient 12, 17–19, 21, 26, 33, 35, 72, 73; *case illus. of* 52–6 *passim*, 59–65 *passim*, 72, 74–5, 83, 88–90 *passim*, 93, 108
social worker's response to 73–5; *case illus. of* 74–5, 79
verbal expression of 18–19
of relatives 38, 40, 73
as a response to mourning 18
reactive 18
despair 25; *case illus. of* 52, 53, 57
detachment from human relationships 92–3; *case illus. of* 85–6, 100
social worker's response to 85–6; *case illus. of* 85–6, 88–90 *passim*
disengagement of self, from life 30–1, 32, 33, 34, 35; *case illus. of* 31
Dominian, J. 3
Doyle, *Sir* Arthur Conan 3
dying work:
of patient:
achievement in 22, 33; *case illus. of* 33
culmination of 27
timing of 34, 36
facilitation of, by social worker *case illus. of* 52–6
initiation of, by social worker 23; *case illus. of* 59–65
interference with 12, 22
problem-solving tasks of 22–36
progress in, inability to make, *case illus. of* 76

social worker's response to 76
psychosocial/emotional stages of
12–21; *case illus. of* 90
term, defined 3
of relatives 39–40
see also acceptance; anger; bargaining; denial; depression; isolation;
terminal care work

Educating for terminal care 9, 43–5,
107, 121–7
programme structure for 122–6
ego 32
endings 44
relevance of terminal care services
to situations involving 5, 128
environmental management 9, 10, 105–6
Erikson, Eric 3
euthanasia 103
relevance of terminal care services
in decision-making regarding 128

Family *see* relatives
fear 14, 25, 26, 48, 50
see also hope and fear, balance of
fear of death:
by caregiver 14, 48, 54
by patient 24, 25, 28, 45–6, 48, 82,
84, 94, 109; *case illus. of* 51
Feifel, H. 113
Foster, Z. P. L. 107, 108, 110–11
free will 32
Freisen, S. R. and Kelly, W. D. 111
friends and neighbours, as caregivers 5
training for 44, 122–7
Fulton, R. 5

Game-playing 13, 14, 22, 23, 37, 48,
95, 96
Garden of Gethsemane 18
giving over *see* control over life, relinquishment of; physical survival
process, reversal of
Glaser, B. G. and Strauss, A. L. 22, 23,
36, 43
God:
anger against 15, 71; *case illus. of* 61
bargaining with 38, 73
blaming 37
commending soul to 34
denial of, *case illus. of* 84–5
faith in xi, 14, 25, 49; *case illus.
of* 31, 89, 92, 93, 94

fear of 26
submitting to will of 32
turning/returning to 32, 35, 39
Goldberg, S. T. 39n
Goldstein, E. G. 105, 107
Good Samaritan, parable of, an
analogy to x
grief 15
grief work:
of patient 39, 40, 67
of relatives, aid of social worker with
104
group social work 104–5
persons who will benefit from 116
guilt feelings:
of patient 18, 26, 33, 37, 83, 94, 99–
100
of relatives 15, 38, 95, 96

Hansen, H. and Knapp, V. S. 104, 105
heaven 31, 89, 90, 94
Hegy, R. 3
hell 31, 33, 84, 94
Henke, Enid, statement by x
Hertzberg, L. J. 112n, 114
Heusinkveltd, K. B. 13, 66
Hineman, J. H. 28
Hinton, J. xi, 32, 39n, 43, 74, 77, 111,
113
home versus hospital, care in 106, 121
hope:
importance of 25, 26, 48, 66, 77, 82,
89; *case illus. of* 62
loss of 27
hope and fear, balance of:
by patient 22, 25–7, 35, 65; *case
illus. of* 26–7, 63, 65, 78–81 *passim*
by relatives 38
social worker's response to 82; *case
illus. of* 78–81 *passim*
hospitalisation, adjustment to, *case
illus. of* 91
Hutchnecker, A. A. 21

Interaction within resource systems,
facilitation of 107, 113
see also interpretative work between
social worker and health disciplines
interpretative work 9, 11, 129
between social worker and health
disciplines 107–8, 109–10, 113, 114,
127; *case illus. of* 108, 114
content of 108
tasks of 110–18